"Sex Smart gets my highest recommendation. It is
empowering guide, and the best book available to
change inhibiting thoughts, feelings, and behaviors stemming from
family-of-origin issues."

> —Barry W. McCarthy, Ph.D.; Professor of Psychology,
> American University; author of *Male Sexual Awareness*
> and *Female Sexual Awareness*

"The exercises offer interesting opportunities for personal growth and
increased understanding of one's sexuality. Must reading for anyone
who seeks to expand their sexual horizon."

> —Howard J. Ruppel, Jr., Ed.D., Ph.D.; Executive
> Director, Society for the Scientific Study of Sexuality
> and the American Association of Sex Educators,
> Counselors, and Therapists

"A fresh look at the complexities of the erotic life. Readers will find the
exercises at the end of each chapter particularly helpful in changing
negative attitudes."

> —David H. Barlow, Ph.D.; Director, Sexuality Research
> and Treatment Program, and Professor, Boston
> University

"Dr. Zoldbrod has an impressive understanding of human
development and the complex interplay between sex and
context—familial, social, and relational.This is a 'user-friendly' book I
would recommend to all clients, gay and straight, since we all lack a
healthy understanding of our sexual development, whether all is going
well or something is going wrong. *Sex Smart* guides us in a warm,
accepting, and knowledgeable way to a fuller integration of our sexual
selves."

> —Claudia Bepko, M.S.W.; family therapist and author of
> *The Responsibility Trap* and *The Heart's Progress*

"Sex Smart is the best explanation of sexuality that we have ever
encountered. Rather than being just another sexual 'cookbook,' it helps
readers examine the origins of their inner messages about sexuality,
allowing a depth of understanding and healing that we believe is
unparalleled in the field."

> —John C. Friel, Ph.D., and Linda Friel, M.A.; licensed
> psychologists and authors of *Adult Children: The
> Secrets of Dysfunctional Families*

"A valuable resource for anyone who wants to understand and explore the root causes of adult sexual intimacy concerns."

—Wendy Maltz, M.S.W.; author of *The Sexual Healing Journey* and *Passionate Hearts*

"With a warm and lively style, Dr. Zoldbrod has condensed a wealth of clinical and scholarly material into an engaging, informative book. I recommend that you read *Sex Smart* if you are seeking to understand your feelings and beliefs about sexuality, how these came to be, and how you might go about changing them. *Sex Smart* is also a great resource for mental health clinicians. The clinical vignettes, practical exercises, and resource lists add to the value of this wonderful book."

—James M. Ellison, M.D., M.P.H.; Associate Clinical Professor in Psychiatry, Harvard Medical School; author of *Integrative Treatment of Anxiety Disorders*

Sex Smart

HOW YOUR CHILDHOOD SHAPED YOUR SEXUAL LIFE AND WHAT TO DO ABOUT IT

Aline P. Zoldbrod, Ph.D.

New Harbinger Publications, Inc.

Distributed in the U.S.A. by Publishers Group West; in Canada by Raincoast Books; in Great Britain by Airlift Book Company; in South Africa by Real Books, Ltd.; in Australia by Boobook; and in New Zealand by Tandem Press.

Cover design by Blue Design.
Edited by Tynan Northrop.
Text design by Michele Waters.

Library of Congress Catalog Card Number: 97-75480
ISBN 1-57224-109-8 Paperback

New Harbinger Publications' Website address: www.newharbinger.com

First printing

Our childhood is stored in our bodies.

—Alice Miller

To the memory of my parents, Monya and Lewis (ZuZu) Zoldbrod—
superb, loving parents, and pretty darned good sex educators.

Contents

Acknowledgments

There are always a lot of people to thank when you write a book.

I would like to thank the many distinguished professionals who took the time to read the manuscript. I am grateful to David Barlow, Ph.D., for his brilliance, his comments, his generosity in taking the time to carefully read and comment, and for the opportunity to present this material to his students. Arnold Lazarus, Ph.D., gets my long-standing appreciation not only for his brilliant contributions to the field, but also for his droll and delightful personal conversations and communications with me. Barry McCarthy, Ph.D., and Claudia Bepko, M.S.W., have been wonderfully supportive, as have Pat Carnes, Ph.D., Gary Brooks, Ph.D., and Ken Minkoff, M.D. Thanks to Barry Reynolds, Ph.D., for some interesting conversations along the way.

Of course, I would never have had the chance to think about these matters if my patients hadn't let me into their lives in such an intimate way. I have been so lucky to have been able to work with them, and I hope that I have helped. I also thank the many professionals, many of whom have become friends, for their confidence in referring patients to me.

I would like to thank my friends, for their support of this project and of me. My lifelong friend, Gerri Schwartz, has been a source of ongoing sustenance, whether she was located in Boston or Austin. I have a memory of riding to Cape Cod with Elaine Aresty, probably three summers ago, when I had the idea for the book but hadn't come up with the theoretical model on which to hang it, and talking it over and over with her. I would also like to acknowledge Francesca Antognini, Ph.D., Jill Vanneman, M.D., Susan Shnidman, Ph.D., Judy Silverstein, Ph.D., James M. Ellison, M.D., and Merle Bombadieri, M.S.W. For anyone I have omitted, I beg your forgiveness.

My friends and colleagues who are authors have to pay a high price for their relationship with me. Walter Clemens, Ph.D., my friend, neighbor, and author of innumerable books on international relations, gets the prize for de-stressing me during times of editorial hysteria. He had a tough-love approach, telling me to get a grip. Carol Frost Vercollone, M.S.W., a longtime friend, also played that role but more in the all-loving therapist mode, even taking calls from me when she was out of town. Thanks, too, to Ellen Rosenberg and Auralie Goodwin, Ph.D.

My children, Monya and Lev Osterweil, are a consistent source of pleasure and fun in my life. Their pride in my career has been long-standing. They see how hard writing is, and they give me the space to do it. When times are tough, they have been known to get themselves invited to friends' houses for sleepovers, partly to preserve my sanity, and partly to preserve theirs. As always, I thank my husband, Larry Osterweil for being there when I need him, and for valuing my creative and therapeutic work. As yet, he hasn't left the house when the going got rough, but he probably wished he could have!

Good health is a tremendous blessing. I have meditated for years on the fact that Strike One, a health club in Burlington, Massachusetts, keeps my body and mind together. I also have to thank my nurse practitioner, Paula Piccolo, who has given me most of my medical care for the last several years. Knowing I have her keeps me feeling secure. I also give a heartfelt thanks to Chris Bent.

I need to thank my whole family. My mother and father, Lewis and Monya Zoldbrod, are both gone now, but their love, empathy, optimism, support, and wisdom stay with me. As a child, I knew how lucky I was to have them as parents. As an adult, and as a therapist who discovers the details of others' lives, I'm amazed at how very fortunate I was.

I am an only child, and my cousins are like my siblings. We tend to share the same world view, for the most part, which is comforting. And they are consistently supportive. I especially would like to thank my cousins Dr. Martha Tolpin, Dr. Bernard Tolpin, Leah Tolpin, Dr. Paul Zolbrod, and Dr. Wilma Austern.

I would like to thank my in-laws, my mother-in-law, Emily Ehrlich, and my aunts, Lilyan Benas and Jeanne Garfinkel (previously known in New York City as the Gorgeous Godnick Girls), for their appreciation of my intellect, their support, their humor, and for Lilyan's food!

I have been so blessed to have worked with the many people at New Harbinger. Thanks to Kristin Beck, and my editors, Farrin Jacobs and Tynan Northrop. The New Harbinger Publications' staff's respect for and cooperation with their authors makes them unusual in the world of publishing.

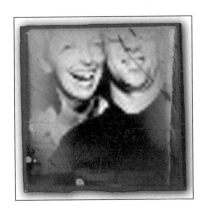

Introduction

Every person has sexual feelings, attitudes and beliefs, but everyone's experience of sexuality is unique because it is processed through an intensely personal experience and public, social sources. It is impossible to understand human sexuality without recognizing its multidimensional nature.

—Robert Masters, Virginia Johnson, and Ralph Kolodny,
On Sex and Human Loving

What Is Sexuality?

What is sexuality? Actually, there is no simple answer to this question, and no sexual expert has put forth a conclusive definition. The dictionary isn't much help: Webster's defines sex as "either of two divisions of organisms distinguished respectively as male and female," or refers to "sexual intercourse." Masters, Johnson, and Kolodny (1988, 5) comment, "The word 'sexuality' generally has a broader meaning, since *it refers to all aspects of being sexual* [emphasis the authors']. Sexuality means a dimension of personality instead of referring to a person's capacity for erotic response alone."

As used in *Sex Smart*, "sexuality" includes a wide range of activities (mental and physical) that may provide sexual delight: a gaze, a conversation, flirting, a dream, a thought, dancing, hugging, kissing, sensual massage, light touching, oral/genital stimulation, digital/genital stimulation, intense merging of two bodies and selves, or intercourse. Although it may be a goal, orgasm is not necessary for sex to be intensely erotic, lusty, and significant, and neither is intercourse.

Why Did You Pick Up This Book?

There are many reasons you may have chosen this book. You may simply be curious about human sexuality. Or you might want to learn about sexual development and the family. *Sex Smart* can add much to your understanding of these issues.

On the other hand, you may have been drawn to this book because you have difficulty feeling good about your own sexuality. Perhaps you have difficulty with many of the sexual activities described above and want to feel better about your sexuality and about yourself as a sexual person. If so, *Sex Smart* will take you on a journey of discovery, helping you to learn why you feel the way you do, and it will provide exercises to help you become a person who is more happy with her sexuality.

Your Family and Your Sexuality

If you picked up this book to change your own sexuality, it is probable that you are mystified about why you feel the way you do sexually. This is understandable, considering that the determinants of your sexuality are not just the explicitly sexual events in your family or personal history (unless you were sexually abused)—they also include the many thematic and daily experiences you had as a child.

Nonsexual Lessons About Sexuality

You've been learning about sexuality since the instant you were born. You found out about it from the way your parents touched you, held you, and diapered you when you were an infant. You were learning about sexuality when you gazed into their eyes, as a tiny baby, and felt (or didn't) a powerful charge of love and connection coming back into your soul. You were learning about sexuality when you broke into your first smile, and your parents smiled and laughed in joy (or didn't). Your parents' affection toward you, as the years went on, taught you whether (or not) you could express affection toward others.

You were learning about sexuality when your parents were encouraged and delighted (or not) by your growing independence—this taught you whether it would be possible to be yourself and still be loved by another person.

Empathy is the ability to understand and feel what another person is feeling. You were getting something very important about sexuality when your parents had empathy for you (or didn't). If your parents didn't have empathy, you may believe that no one can really understand you, so it isn't worth trying to talk about how you feel or what you want.

You were learning about sexuality when you felt (or didn't feel) your parents' deep concern and attachment to you. If they paid attention to your upsets, you learned to trust. If they were neglectful, you learned suspicion.

Your parents' reaction to your gender was important, too. Either you felt they were glad that you were a girl/boy and that you made a very cute little girl/boy, or you felt confusion and/or their disappointment about your gender. You also learned significant lessons about sexuality and gender from the way your parents treated each other. If the male/female relationship you saw modeled by your parents was abusive, you might not feel good about being the same gender as the abuser—or the same gender as the victim.

Your sexuality was affected profoundly by the way your parents handled power, between themselves and in the way they disciplined you. If there was violence in your family, it stunted your sexual growth, because you now subconsciously associate intimacy, control, and danger.

And your parents had a huge impact on your sexual life by the way they encouraged or discouraged you developing social skills. If they were overprotective, or isolated you, or didn't help you to learn how to get along with other people as a child, they created a deficit that you will have to remedy as an adult. None of these lessons was explicitly sexual, yet all of them were crucial. *Sex Smart* takes an in-depth look into these nonsexual aspects of your sexual evolution.

What Is Sexual Socialization?

Most of what you may already have read in trying to figure out what makes you tick, sexually, describes sexual socialization (what you were taught about how to be a sexual human being) in terms of what your family *literally* taught you about sex. Some excellent books talk about different family sexual environments ranging from families which are completely inhibited about discussing sex, to families which are appropriate and open in discussing sexuality, to families where things are overly seductive or there is outright sexual abuse. These overtly sexual aspects of your family are important factors in who you turned out to be, sexually, but they are only a piece of the whole picture.

Dr. Helen Calderone (Calderone and Johnson 1981) clearly defines the key elements of a child's sexual socialization:

- recognition and acceptance of the pleasure factor

- careful and consistent socialization for privacy and responsibility, and appropriateness of time, place, and person

- continuing education about the nature and purposes of sex

- building self-esteem about the goodness of all the child's human endowments, including sex

- putting the child in charge of its body and all of its functions

Does this sound like your own sexual socialization? Maybe it was, or maybe not. Perhaps your family wasn't open and flexible enough to take the tips offered by experts in child sexual development. Many of these books assume a healthy, open, loving family structure, and high-functioning parents who have a lot of energy, time, and the commitment to devise the best way to raise their children to become healthy, responsible sexual adults. Most books advise parents on gender role issues, how to talk openly about sexuality, or how to be "askable" parents. For flourishing families that are comfortable about sexuality, this advice and direction would be enough.

But many of you have come from households that weren't this healthy. If you grew up in a family where your parents didn't feel good about themselves sexually (or in general), or where the children weren't treated well, even if you had been taught these "correct" messages about being sexual, you would discard the carefully selected sexual information fed to you. Instead, the constant hidden emotional messages about sex and relationships—fear, distrust, shame, or disgust—would be learned.

Probably the most important way in which your family affected you was the lessons you learned about whether or not you want to be close to another person, to join in relationship. This creates your basic motivation for sex. As discussed by Steve Levine, M.D. (1988), part of what we usually think of as sexual desire is not just the physical drive to be sexual—it also includes the wish to act sexually, and the motivation to be sexual with a specific person: "the desire for desire" (Rosen and Lieblum 1987, 148).

What Is "Healthy" Sexuality?

Sexuality is such a complicated wonder that there is no generally accepted definition of what "healthy" sexuality is, even among experts. Your own ideas might vary from someone else's, according to your age, your politics, your religion, your gender, your sexual orientation, or your culture. The point of *Sex Smart* isn't to make you accept someone else's definition of healthy sexuality; it is to help you define and actualize your own sexual wishes and ideals.

If you can grow enough to experience and appreciate the whole display of sexual enjoyments, such as the ones mentioned on page 2, I guarantee that this concept of healthy sexuality will give you pleasure throughout your entire life, through illness, through sorrows, and into old age.

My ultimate hope is that you, with the help of this book, will be able to express your sexual self fully—at the most intense, to be able to joyfully lose your boundaries in a sexual trance with a person to whom you are emotionally committed.

Why Do People Have Sex?

People have sex and behave in sexual ways for a whole host of reasons. Sexual experts don't even agree about whether or not certain uses of sexuality are better or more healthy than others. But they do agree that sex is a natural, healthy part of living. You need to decide for yourself which motivating forces you like and dislike.

According to Robert Crooks and Karla Baur (1993, 198), people behave sexually:

- as a validation of deep intimacy within a relationship

- as a way of getting to know someone

- for reproduction

- to reduce sexual tension

- as a way of experiencing new feelings, excitement, risk

- for a recreational pastime

- to alleviate feelings of insecurity

- to prove manhood or womanhood

- to please someone

- to persuade someone to care

- to experience the power to attract others

- to avenge earlier rejections by enticing partners and turning them down

Milestones in Sexual Development

Sex Smart is based on a simple model. This model describes different stages—the most important things that needed to happen in your sexual development in order for you to feel comfortable letting go and experiencing deep sexual pleasure with a loved partner. I have called these stages the "Milestones in Sexual Development" (see appendix A). They include:

- being loved

- being touched

- receiving empathy

- learning to trust

- learning how to relax and be soothed by the person you trust

- developing a good body image

- becoming comfortable in your gender identity

- developing self-esteem

- knowing how to handle power well, and feeling that you own yourself

- having permission to explore yourself, your body, and your sexual feelings

- learning how to develop social skills

Adolescent issues:

- integrating masturbation or sexual fantasy into your life in a healthy way

- separating from your parents

- being able to be in a loving, sexual relationship with another person

Sexual development is unbelievably complex and somewhat idiosyncratic. No one could possibly make the perfect, definitive, one-size-fits-all model of family issues in sexual development. The important issues in your household may not have unfolded in exactly the order of the chapters in this book. But in any case, you need to examine each stage and investigate, for yourself, any correlations in your own personal development.

One of the problems with a lot of the fix-it-yourself sex therapy articles in magazines, and even many of the self-help therapy books, is that they ignore sexual problems caused by very early events with love, touch, empathy, trust, fear, and disturbed power relationships. These first stumbling blocks affect millions and millions of readers—any of you who grew up in a neglectful, alcohol-or-drug-ridden, violent, cold, or unempathic home. It can be painful to admit that you grew up in a neglectful or violent home, but it is important to be honest with yourself. In appendix B on page 239, you will find a superb checklist by Ellen Ratner (1990) that will help you screen for such early issues. Please complete this checklist before you proceed with the rest of *Sex Smart*.

What This Book Covers—And What It Doesn't

Sex Smart has much to offer readers who want to actualize themselves sexually, but it will hold the key to solving some readers' problems better than others. *Sex Smart* will be especially helpful if you are confused because you aren't comfortable sexually, and you came from a "good" home with basically decent, loving, responsible parents where there was no sexual abuse. *Sex Smart* also has a lot to teach you if you came from a "not so good" or "bad" home and want to explore its impact.

In addition, *Sex Smart* is one of the only books that describes the effects of nonsexual family violence on adult sexuality; a whole chapter is devoted to this topic. If you grew up in a violent family, please read chapter 11 after you read this introduction and have completed Ratner's checklist (page 239), then go on to the rest of the book. If, on the other hand, you were abused sexually, you should first explore your sexuality by reading a book written for survivors of sexual abuse, *then* read *Sex Smart*. If you have come from a very traumatic background, it would be best to read this book *with your therapist*. Some of the contents are explicit and may trigger you in upsetting ways.

For some readers, *Sex Smart* has more severe limitations, because certain sexual problems are based on other realities, not in past family experience. This book does not speak to sexual problems based in societal prejudice. Any of you who are physically unattractive or who have physical disabilities or disfigurements know that no matter what your personal worth, and no matter how loving and open your family has been about sexuality, it can be difficult to find a partner for love and sexual connection.

Sometimes, sexual problems can have medical causes. Certain illnesses (for instance, diabetes) and certain medications (such as antihypertensives and antidepressants) have sexual side effects. Before you assume that your issues are psychological, see your physician for an evaluation of whether or not your problem might be organic (see also appendix C).

In addition, your sexual motivation for being in any relationship will depend on your feelings for the other person. This aspect of sexuality is outside the scope of *Sex Smart,* though you may find the checklist in appendix D helpful for determining what relationship factors to look for.

While this book describes aspects of sexual development relevant to bisexual and homosexual people, it is not definitive in that regard. Researchers and clinicians have only now begun to break through their heterosexual bias, and there isn't all that much information out there yet on normal sexual development for bisexual and homosexual people. While *Sex Smart* attempts to account for different lifestyles and cultures, it may not have succeeded. Your comments, wisdom, and suggestions are welcome. Please write to:

Aline Zoldbrod / Sex Smart Feedback
C/O New Harbinger Publications
5674 Shattuck Avenue
Oakland, CA 94609

Where to Begin

Keeping a journal can be extremely helpful in assessing your sexual development as well as monitoring your progress toward healthy adult sexuality. Choose a notebook or three-ring binder and divide it into eleven sections—one for each chapter of *Sex Smart.* Starting with chapter 1, use the list of questions at the beginning of each chapter as a guide to determine if the sexual issues discussed in that chapter pertain to you. If so, you may want to write your answers to the questions in your journal before proceeding with the chapter.

As you read through the book, case examples of problems that occurred in different stages of other people's lives will hopefully help you identify patterns in your own life. Whenever you make such connections, write them down in your journal in the appropriate section.

After reading each chapter, write some notes in your journal on how the themes discussed in the chapter relate to your sexual development. And be sure to do the exercises at the end of each relevant chapter!

Your Road Map

Think of *Sex Smart* as your personal road map—and your journal as your travel diary. Hopefully, with each chapter, you'll be able to figure out what went wrong in each area of your sexual development and address it. By the end of the book, you will most likely have discovered that your sexual block or difficulty wasn't caused by an isolated event or doesn't fall into just one of the chapter areas—it is the result of many incidents, behaviors, and different developmental stages. Your *Sex Smart* journal will reflect your new understanding of your own personal path, clarifying the most important issues for you, and pave the road to your expanded sexuality.

Exercise

Define Your Goals for Healthy Sexuality

To help define your own goals, go through the following list and put a "G" next to each of the goals you want to accomplish. If you don't agree that an item should be a goal, cross it out entirely. Finally, put a check mark next to the goals you have already attained.

_____ I equate touching and being touched with pleasure.

_____ I associate touching with love.

_____ I have a sense of personal safety.

_____ I have the self-confidence to reach out and make contact with a person to whom I am attracted.

_____ I have the basic social skills to form an emotionally intimate relationship with a friend.

_____ I feel safe asking for what I want and need within an emotionally intimate relationship.

_____ I am able to reciprocate emotionally, to meet the needs of my closest friends and loved ones.

_____ I am able to feel trust in a person who has basically been consistently fair, kind, and loving toward me.

_____ I am able to relax and feel pleasure in an appropriate sexual situation with a trusted and loved person.

_____ I am able to commit within a relationship.

_____ I am able to feel empathy for the person(s) I love.

_____ I don't have inappropriate guilt and shame about myself, my body, or my sexual feelings.

_____ I feel that I own my own body.

_____ I feel able to sexually explore and pleasure my own body.

_____ I am my own sexual expert: I know what turns me on.

_____ I am able to ask for the specific kinds of sexual touches and activities that I like.

_____ I can gratify my sexual urges without hurting or using others.

_____ It gives me sexual pleasure to give sexual pleasure to the person I love.

_____ I only have safe sex.

_____ I can experience sensations in the moment.

_____ I am not afraid to turn my body over to the sexual experience, to let go, or to go into a sexual trance.

_____ I have the right to be an autonomous sexual being.

_____ I accept my body, with all of its imperfections.

_____ I accept my own gender, sexual orientation, and sexual identity.

_____ I live within my own ethical and moral value system, when it comes to sex.

_____ I have the capacity to forgive my past sexual blunders and misdeeds.

_____ I am able to try new sexual experiences.

_____ I am able to ask for sexual contact from others and I am able to refuse it, when others ask and I don't want it.

_____ I am able to ask for help when I have sexual problems.

As you read this book and decide how you want to change, keep the goals you have indicated in mind.

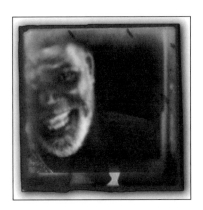

Chapter 1

The Touch of Love

The young mother approaches her baby with outstretched arms. He hears her coming and immediately turns his head toward her. His eyes lock onto hers and they both smile faintly. He throws his arms up toward her as she reaches down and swoops him up. She holds him up and stares into his eyes with the look of joy, excitement, and adoration. They both begin cooing and babbling. She serenades him with the rhythmic, high pitched but low and tender voice of the universal baby talk. Then she cuddles him to her soft, warm body and begins rocking him back and forth, intermittently cooing, gurgling, babbling, singing, laughing, and sometimes "tearing up" with joy.

What is going on here? You know immediately what it all means, the mother knows, and even the one-year-old baby knows, all without ever uttering one meaningful word. The mother and baby are loving each other. Putting it as precisely as we can . . . the mother and her son are adoring *each other completely in the* primal scene of loving.

—Jack D. Douglas and Freda Cruse Atwell, *Love, Intimacy, and Sex*

♦ **Do you associate touching and love?**

♦ **Do you associate touching and safety?**

♦ **Does it make you feel secure to make eye contact with someone you like or love?**

♦ **Do you enjoy the sights, sounds, smells, and tastes of making love?**

A secure, loving attachment to your primary caretaker—usually your mother—is your first testing ground to learn love. It is within that relationship that most of us discover the many small behaviors and feelings which we ultimately need in order to be able to enjoy the dissolution of boundaries which occurs in ecstatic sexual union.

When you are examining your feelings about being a sexual person, you should first notice how you feel about giving and receiving touch. Touching isn't sexual *per se*, but touch is the foundation upon which your ability to enjoy sexuality is built; it is vital to loving and to sexual expression. To have skin contact with a partner and to feel the warmth of his (or her) body remains an essential component of many kinds of love relationships.

What does touching mean in your family of origin? Does touching mean love, help, comfort, fun, pleasure? Is it easy for you to express your loving feelings through touching another person? Or does gentle physical contact feel unfamiliar and strange? Does sensual touch feel bad, bringing up memories of guilt? Does any kind of touch bring a startled response, or memories of pain and fear?

If you were lucky, you grew up in a family in which love was expressed through touch. You associate touch with caring, safety, comfort, and relaxation. You feel confident using touch to express wishes for more intimacy or a desire for more or less physical contact. You naturally use touch to diffuse anger, and to smooth over disagreements.

When you are on the receiving end, your associations to your partner's touches are good ones. Gentle touch makes you feel cared for, safe, important, and valued. When you want to, you can let touch lead you down the pathway to sexual ecstasy.

Ironically, touch is so basic to sexuality and yet there are millions and millions of people whose enjoyment of sexuality is hampered by problems with physical contact. They don't feel comfortable, natural, relaxed, or safe giving or receiving touch.

Some people come from loving families who didn't touch, so touching was never linked to love. Other people come from loving-but-anxious families, so touch is linked with anxiety. In some families, the meaning of touch has been distorted by neglect, violence, or sexual abuse (see chapters 10 and 11).

I feel that if I had one thing I could change about my childhood, not being touched would be it. I don't think there is anything more isolating. Plus it makes you feel like you are a leper or something, because all around you people are touching each other. In books, people are touching each other, too. But no one is touching you . . .

—Sandy, 23

I think I was affected negatively by the fact that my mother was emotionally responsive to us as children, but not physically. She wasn't comfortable with physical attention. She would tell me to "stop being mushy" if I hugged her too long.

—Trina, 35

And I had this dream that I was in your office and you were stroking my hair, which is something that an uncle of mine did to me one time when I was eleven or twelve and needed it. And the feeling of being comforted was so strong (and so unique to me) that it stuck with me.

—Greta, 49

The Benefits of Touch

Suki, a four-and-a-half-year-old girl, jumped onto her mother's lap, wrapped her arms around her, sucked her mom's nose and licked her ears. Her mother, who loves touch, hugged the child back, kissed her, and laughed.

We humans learn to love not by instruction, but by being loved. In psychologist Harry Harlow's famous experiments with baby monkeys (1965, 1969), Harlow found that the need for physical attachment and comfort superseded the need for food.

Anthropologist Ashley Montagu, Ph.D. (1971), looked at the role of touch in the development of animals and humans. He proved that humans have to undergo certain kinds of tactile experiences in order to develop normally. In all sorts of mammals, study after study which Montagu reviewed proved that touching by the mother animal was crucial to behavioral development. Animals which were gentled by their mother were soft-hearted, unexcitable animals. Lack of gentling produced fearful, excitable young ones.

Babies are soothed by touching and warmth (Ainsworth 1978, 1982). Studies of infants in orphanages (Bowbly 1971–79) have shown that unless human infants are touched lovingly by their caretakers, they become depressed and may die.

The Pleasures of Having a Body

"Sexuality" isn't just intercourse or genital contact. It begins with a basic, instinctive response of pleasure to touch. At best, parents impart a basic optimism about the body—the child's body as an entity, and bodies interacting together. Look around you and watch the parents you see in crowds, or at parks. There are huge differences in the ways parents touch their infants and children and in the messages children are given about their bodies.

Some children are just lucky enough to grow up in families where affectionate touch is as available as air for breathing, and bodies are seen as vehicles for fun. People who grow up with a lot of love and affection tend to feel very comfortable and contented with sexuality as adults.

Some people have wonderful memories of being touched throughout their childhood, when physical contact is used to soothe, to connect, for affection, or for play. They remember jumping into their father's (or mother's) arms at parks, or "dancing" while standing on top of a parent's legs while that parent moved around, carrying them, or actually dancing grown-up style with their parent at a special event.

When a parent takes a child in her arms and comforts her when she is upset, or physically hurt, that parent is teaching the child the fundamental positive ingredient of sexuality. When a father wakes up a child in the morning by quietly talking to him and rubbing his back, he is teaching him about sexuality. When parents, with watchful eyes, encourage a child to jump on a trampoline, or to climb and swing on a jungle gym, you could even make the case that these parents are teaching the child about sexuality. From a young age, all these children associate touch with love and soothing, and they associate their own bodies with play, delight, relaxation, excitement, love, fun, competence, pleasure.

Children who associate touch with love, in turn, touch their parents lovingly and empathically. When they are still tiny, these children then begin using touch to show love and caring for others.

A little girl of fifteen months comes up to her mother, who is in the early stage of labor with the girl's sibling. When the mother grimaces in pain, the little girl comes up to her, kisses her, and says,

"Poor mommy." This tiny child has already become comfortable expressing love and caring with touch.

Culture and Touch

How touch was handled in your family depends, in part, on your ethnic background. Different ethnic groups have dissimilar sets of values and behavior. For instance, Greek families lovingly touch their young children quite frequently (Welts 1982); Portugese children tend to be touched affectionately from infancy only until school age (Moitoza 1982); and Irish families do not express their love through touching (McGoldrick 1982).

North American culture, as a whole, isn't very touch-feely. Compared to people of some other nationalities, we in the United States are a bunch of cold fish. In one study of friends in a coffee shop, American pals were found to touch each other an average of twice an hour, while French friends touched 110 times and Puerto Rican friends 180 times (Alfvin 1995).

Loving Eye Contact: Another Kind of Touch

My mother was a very cold woman, very cold. I can't ever even remember seeing her look at me and smile. I'm still afraid of women. There are times when I want to reach out and connect, and I can't do it. I just withdraw. I can't make the first step toward contact.

—Jim, 46

Take some time, now, to think about the kind of eye contact shared by members of your family, because eye contact is a kind of nonphysical touch. It is in the parent-child bond where you probably first learned the "look of love." However, in some families, loving eye contact between parent and child was missing.

In the primal scene of love described at the beginning of this chapter, the baby and the mother gaze at each other. In fact, according to Douglas and Atwell (1988), it is common for a mother who loves her baby securely to pick the baby up, hold its face directly in front of hers, so that she can focus her eyes fully on the baby's eyes, and look into those eyes with complete intimacy for as long as twenty seconds or more—this is the longest period of unblinking eye-fixation found in human experience. Douglas and Atwell comment, "She and the baby are looking into each other's souls. They are *communing* with each other, expressing and receiving adoration, love, and the sense of self" (p. 58).

In adult relationships, Dr. Helen E. Fisher (1993) describes the gaze as the most striking human courting ploy. According to Dr. Fisher, in Western societies, where eye contact between the sexes is permitted, flirting men and women often stare intently at potential mates for about two or three seconds, during which their pupils often dilate—a sign of extreme interest. Afterward, the starer looks away.

With enough experience in loving communion with your mother (or other adoring parent), in infancy and beyond, you automatically learn to look at other people to whom you are attracted with a smile. (Often this happens so subconsciously that you let the other person know your interest even before you, yourself, are consciously aware of it.) Without the early experience of receiving adoring gazes, reaching out to others to make intellectual, emotional, or romantic connections probably feels too risky.

> Steve, a single man, came into therapy to work on his difficulty attracting women and starting relationships. When talking about his futile attraction to a woman in his church group, and how he couldn't just look at her and smile, so that she would know he was interested, he said, "Smiling at another person doesn't feel natural . . . . I think if I really look at her a lot, she'll punch me, or turn me in to the cops."
>
> Steve's discomfort with eye contact was a major ingredient in his inability to connect with a partner. As it turns out, his mother had spent his early years more in love with a bottle of alcohol than she was with him. She neglected him in his infancy and didn't spend time engaged with him face-to-face, gazing at him, playing with him, or singing or talking to him.
>
> Because Steve's mother hadn't adored him, eye contact with a woman to whom he was attracted felt dangerous and unfamiliar. In therapy, Steve soon figured out that because he wanted attention but was fearful of rejection, he wasn't able to make good eye contact with women. Women didn't trust him. This led to potential partners actually rejecting him, further frightening him. Steve had to learn to risk making eye contact with others, practicing in the safest situations for small amounts of time, then building towards

making eye contact for longer periods of time and in less safe situations.

Pleasure or Anxiety?: Styles of Attachment

Bill came into sex therapy with his wife, Vanessa. Bill had always felt comfortable with sexuality, but Vanessa had never been interested. When looking into what each of them had learned in their family about being sexual, they found that Bill's mother was very affectionate, while Vanessa's family had been very cold.

With pleasure, Bill recalled an intense memory he had about his mother's belief in touching. At age ten, an uncle was visiting their house. Bill was resting on the couch, next to his mother, and he was leaning back into his mother's arm and resting his head on her full breasts. The uncle criticized him for being too old for this. Bill's mother jumped right in and told the uncle, in no uncertain terms, that this was perfectly all right and that she was glad they had such a close relationship. Bill identifies his mother's openness with touching as an important building block in his love of sex.

Recent research supports what many sex therapists see in their practices: that when people grow up in families which fail to link touch to pleasure, relaxation, and love, sexual problems result. Psychologists Shaver, Hazan, and Bradshaw (1984) found that babies, in their first years of life, adopt three different ways of relating: secure, anxious, or avoidant—depending on how caregivers treated them. Secure babies see their mothers as available and interested. They feel free to explore the world. Anxious infants see their mothers as sporadic caregivers and are always in a worried quest to win their mother's love. Avoidant babies see their mothers as physically and emotionally rejecting, and learn to turn off their needs and feelings as a result.

Styles of attachment as infants seem to be related to adults' ways of relating to other people and to their subjective feelings about their sex lives. Secure adults found it relatively easy to get close to others. They enjoyed nearly all physical and sexual contact, from cuddling to oral sex. They were willing to experiment sexually, but to do so in the context of a continuing relationship. They were unlikely to engage in one-night stands or to have sex outside of their primary relationship.

Avoidant adults tended to become less invested in relationships and tended to be lonelier. They demonstrated less enjoyment of all physical, as opposed to sexual, contact. That result fits well with infancy researchers finding that the parents of avoidant children disliked close physical contact.

Anxious adults liked the physical, nurturing aspects of the relationship, but were not as thrilled with sexual expression. In their interactions with other adults, they scored low on sensitivity and high on compulsive caregiving.

There Is No Substitute for Touch

There are plenty of excellent, otherwise adoring, consistent, and concerned parents out in the world who feel unable to use touch to express their love for their children. If your parents were like Sylvia's mother, you might find it difficult to connect touching, love, and sexuality.

> Sylvia grew up alone with only her mother. Her father had abandoned them when Sylvia was only two years old. Her mother, Joan, loved her very much, and was a very responsible caretaker in almost every way. Unfortunately, she didn't like to touch.
>
> When Sylvia wanted to hug and kiss her mother, Joan asked her "not to be mushy." When Sylvia wanted to climb into her mother's lap, Joan told her that that would mess up her work clothes, and then she wouldn't be able to go into the city and make the money they needed to survive.
>
> But Sylvia knew her mother loved her, and she grew up feeling good about herself in many ways. Joan taught Sylvia how to take care of the house and be responsible for getting dinner on, leaving Sylvia elaborate instructions for every step of the preparation. Sylvia always did as she was told, and Joan frequently bought her little trinkets to show her approval for Sylvia's responsible behavior. Sylvia still cherishes the set of Russian nesting dolls her mother once brought her home, as a reward for her helpful behavior during a particularly difficult week.
>
> As an adult, Sylvia has trouble in relationships with men. She is not comfortable expressing herself through touch or sexuality. She expresses her love in exactly the way she was taught to: she takes care of her boyfriends by ironing their clothes, packing their lunches and their luggage for trips, and organizing life for them both. She keeps the house spotless. But because Joan didn't link touch and love in Sylvia's childhood, Sylvia can't relax and get comfortable with being sexual, so she avoids sex as much as she

can. Sylvia cannot understand why all of her boyfriends eventually leave her, despite the many ways in which she shows her love for them.

If you feel uncomfortable with being sexual, like Sylvia, and your parents were basically good, self-sacrificing, loving parents who weren't comfortable with touch, it may be painful, or guilt-producing, to let yourself admit that your parents weren't saints. But don't, as Sylvia did, avoid facing the issue that affection and sexuality make you feel uncomfortable. Instead, work on increasing your comfort with touch, and use the exercises at the end of this chapter as a guide.

Turning Up One's Nose

Ben was dragged into marital therapy by his wife Elise, after fifteen years of marriage. She complained about his "meat and potatoes" style of lovemaking. "Ben hates all of the sights, smells, or touches of lovemaking," complained Elise. "He doesn't like to lie around and cuddle, is always complaining that I need to take a shower, even when I am perfectly clean, and he can't stand to touch my vagina. He never makes a sound when we make love."

As we explored his history, Ben became aware that his mother, Nina, was extremely fastidious, almost phobic, physically. He recalled that he and his sister used to laugh about his mother's bathroom habits. Growing up, when his mother left the bathroom, there never was any evidence that she had ever had any bodily functions at all: no smell of gas, no trace of urine, no used sanitary tampons in the bathroom. He and his sister used to wonder how she did it!

Elise recalled watching her mother-in-law coming to help after their first child was born, and changing the baby for them. Nina went at the task in a perfunctory, almost rote way. She wrinkled up her nose at the smell of the dirty diaper, and threw it away by using only two fingers, in order to touch it as little as possible. She cleaned the baby thoroughly, and then rediapered her as quickly as she could, not taking any time to play with the baby, or kiss her naked skin. The task accomplished, she proudly handed a clean-again baby back to Elise.

As Ben and Elise told these stories, they began to understand the source of Ben discomforts with bodily sights, sounds, tastes, and smells. Ben decided to take some time to reprocess and change the negative lessons he had learned about touching, sights, smells, and sounds.

It isn't easy to make the kinds of changes Ben needed to make. Whatever way you make love grew out of what has been comfortable. The first step often is a new sense of self-observation, a new awareness of your own embarrassment with the earthiness of sexual contact. You might notice that you are wondering for the first time *why* certain activities you disdain are repulsive to you, rather than simply avoiding them. Initially, realizing your profound shyness will make you feel less adequate sexually, not better. But the more you read, think, look at, and experiment with new ways of being physical, the more your sexual repetoire will grow.

Loving but Anxious

Because subconscious associations to touch are so powerful in determining adult sexual response, growing up with loving parents who were anxious in their physical caretaking can create sexual problems. When parents are overconcerned emotionally, and also very clingy physically, touch comes to mean suffocation and anxiety rather than fun, comfort, or relaxation.

Zack and Greta entered marriage therapy and presented some issues about sexuality as well. Greta was very much in love with Zack, and he felt the same way about her. Verbally, he was wonderfully sensitive and supportive. He was tender with their children, and able to enjoy being physical with them in a playful, loving way. But Greta complained that Zack seemed to pull away from her whenever she wanted to be affectionate.

Zack was puzzled by his own reactions. He was attracted to Greta physically, and loved her. Yet his subconscious reaction, if she reached out to grab him, or wanted to spoon in bed with him, was to run or push her away.

After months of exploration, Zack finally made the connection, which went back to his parents. Both were loving, but anxious. His father was more distant, but his mother's caretaking and touching had an anxious and intrusive quality. Zack saw that his association to Greta's holding him was the same feeling of suffocation he got in his family, when his mother's overconcern and compulsive physical caretaking and touching made him want to escape.

Zack also realized that he didn't have the same reaction when his children wanted to cuddle because they were so small, relative to him, that he never had concerns about being suffocated or controlled.

Neglectful, Violent, or Abusive

Families where parents physically and emotionally neglect or abuse children, and families where the parents are physically violent toward each other produce children whose associations to touch and love are deeply damaged.

John is terrified of connecting to another person. Still a virgin, in his fifties, he has never been in a serious relationship, although he is well liked at work and by the parishioners at his church.

John is the third child of four boys. John's mother tried to make do in her life with her alcoholic husband. She grew so depressed that her capacity to nurture her children was severely limited. By the time John was born, she didn't have much energy left. John was a "good baby" who didn't cry much. His mother left him in the crib much of the time, because she was busy with his older sibs. Her "caretaking" was very haphazard. As John got older, his mother left his older brothers in charge of him. He remembers a time that he was smashed in the face by a hardball at a game, and when he went to his brother with his bloodied face and broken glasses, he just laughed at him.

John never linked touch with love, and he learned that no one could be trusted. Naturally, making a sexual connection to another person feels terrifying to John. The few times that a woman has tried to be affectionate, he became frightened and confused and pulled away. He longs for a relationship, but is too petrified to initiate anything. He doesn't believe that he is lovable and is terribly afraid of the pain of being disappointed if he becomes dependent on anyone.

Growing up in a home with any kind of violence changes one's sexual associations in still another way: Human touch comes to be associated with physical danger. It is not uncommon for men and women from violent homes to have a total inability to close their eyes and relax. Trust in the physical safety of the world has been broken.

If you have realized that you or your partner's attitudes toward touching and sexuality has been severely distorted by a violent, abusive, or neglectful family, read chapter 11 before you go on to chapter 3.

There Is Hope

If you grew up in a home where your parents never touched you tenderly and appropriately, becoming comfortable with touch as an adult may seem like a difficult, if not impossible, undertaking. But the good news is that learning to like touching and being touched is something that you *can* do at any point in life.

If you are in a loving and safe relationship with another person who cares about your welfare and growth and who is mature enough to give you a vacation from pressure for genital contact, you have a perfect situation in which to learn some of the joys of nonsexual touch.

> Betty and Sam had been married for six years. Although they had had a wonderful marriage, with mutual respect and love, Betty had never enjoyed lovemaking. She couldn't relax, and she never felt sexual pleasure. She just had sex with Sam as part of her "wifely" duty. She commented that she saw her body "as a means to carry my head around." They decided, at Sam's urging, to enter sexual therapy.
>
> In discussing their sexual histories, it became clear that Betty's family was rather critical and cold. In addition, the parents very rarely touched the children lovingly. They were serious workers, who believed that if they didn't drink alcohol and always kept their children clean and fed, they were being excellent parents.
>
> In sexual therapy, it took many, many weeks before Betty and Sam could take time off from their chores and relax enough to even *try* sensual, nongenital touching. At first when they did it, Betty felt strange about it. But after she got used to it, Betty began talking about how special it makes her feel to be touched, when Sam spends a lot of time on her. She realized that this was the first time

she really felt that special to anyone and had enjoyed the touching and how relaxing it had been.

They came in after a week of vacation. During the past two weeks, they had been doing the sensual touching and had begun to touch genitals. There was something different about the way they were talking about it. Betty was talking about how relaxing it felt, but not talking about how it was sexually exciting.

Sam was expressing some anxiety that he was "doing something wrong." Betty kept saying that Sam wasn't doing anything wrong, that it all felt good, relaxing, and that she was finally getting to the point of accepting that she deserved to be touched like this. It was obvious that Sam was upset that Betty wasn't turned on sexually in any way. At the same time, Betty was taking much more pleasure in touching Sam and giving him pleasure. Sam said something about them being on a plateau.

Something else was going on that had to be integrated: Betty was beginning to feel the pleasure in her body of being loved in a physical way (not a sexual way, yet) that she had missed in her childhood.

Betty spoke excitedly: "Yes, that's exactly right. This is what is going on. I'm finally feeling, 'Gee, this really is happening to me. Someone really is touching me like this. I really am getting these touches and hugs.' It is almost as if I am picking up a piece of the puzzle and fitting it in, when I didn't even know that a piece was missing."

Betty said that sometimes, she was actually having an out-of-body experience, where she was looking down at herself and saying, "Wow! This really is happening to you. Someone is touching you like this."

All of what she was feeling from the tenderness and the touching was tied in her mind to her self-worth. It didn't have any sexual connotations yet, really. In fact, Betty was tapping into a very powerful knowledge, but a sad one, too, that this experience was one she needed in her childhood but had entirely missed. And while she didn't actually feel sad right as he was touching her, she felt sad at the loss afterward.

So Betty was going back, developmentally, and learning how to link touch with love. And just like loving touch shouldn't/ wouldn't be linked with adult genital sexuality for a child, it wasn't with Betty yet. She needed to take some time to let herself have this new physical experience of being loved—of having physical pleasure given to her—without it being sexual, yet.

And at the same time, since love and touch were being linked in a new way for her, she was touching Sam in a new way. Sam now reported that she was coming over to him, routinely, and touching him on the back, or giving him hugs, during the day. She had never done that before. And even though she couldn't be genital yet herself, Betty was enjoying touching Sam's penis and giving him genital pleasure in a new way now.

Sam tolerated feeling left out emotionally for several more months as Betty thought about her family's attitude toward touch and felt a new sadness. Sam also had to take care of many of his own needs, sexually, for that time period. They spent a lot of time together taking massages and baths together.

Sam began to wonder whether Betty would ever feel turned on, or whether she would just stay at this stage where she felt physical pleasure and relaxation. But he was a wonderfully patient man, and it paid off.

After a few months of learning about touch, Betty's therapist started her on exercises to discover her own abilities to give herself sexual pleasure. Betty did this new homework, and quickly, she began to integrate her new ability to relax and make the emotional connection between touch and love. After about sixteen months of sexual therapy, Sam and Betty reported having sexual passion in their marriage for the first time.

The dramatic change which occurred in Betty's feelings about herself and her sexuality was amazing. The most important ingredient in their success was their deeply loving and respectful emotional connection to each other. Sam managed to put most of his hurt and upset feelings into words. He didn't withhold, sulk, get angry, or punish Betty when she needed to withhold intercourse in order to explore her own feelings. He put his sense of being left out of her emotional life into words, too, and thus avoided increasing the emotional distance which had temporarily been created in their relationship.

Not all connections are as safe and as strong as Betty and Sam's. If you and your lover have a relationship where communication is a problem, or at least one of you is full of tension, resentment, or has problems regarding power and control, then you will need to strengthen your nonsexual relationship first, before you go on to changing your feelings about sexuality.

The Importance of Nongenital Touch

Some younger men with strong sex drives do not realize their general discomfort with receiving touch, since they define being sexual as penile penetration, and their erectile response is strong. If their partners do not complain about getting enough nongenital touching before intercourse, the sexual routine may not include much intimate, nonpenetrating touch. But learning more of the pleasures of whole-body touch may become crucial to men in the midlife years, when sexual drive diminishes somewhat, and automatic erections stop occurring. Many men haven't read much about the normal changes which occur with age and they panic. They believe that they should be able to be aroused instantaneously, and it isn't as easy anymore. In midlife, much to their surprise, being touched by their partner becomes an important route to sexual arousal. Thus, sometimes it isn't until middle age that problems or discomforts with touch become evident for men.

Women's bodies function differently from men's, and throughout women's lifespan, the full sexual arousal important for orgasm usually depends on a period of nongenital touch. So, women who are not comfortable with nongenital touch often complain of lack of arousal.

Exercises

Strategies for Increasing Your Comfort with Touching and Being Touched

Positive and Negative Associations to Touch

Make a copy of the following list of good and bad feelings about each. Date it and circle the feelings that apply to how *you* feel about touch.

Positive	**Negative**
Safety	Fear
Caring	Controlling
Warmth	Out of control
Soothing	Pain
Love	Awkward

Positive	Negative
Pleasure	Numb
Relaxation	Tense / anxiety
Fun	Guilt
Softness	Startle response
Good memories	Bad memories
Comfort	Discomfort
Normal	Weird
Help	Danger
Connection	Confusion
I'm worth touching	What does this mean?
Calming	Jumpy
Indulgence	Is this proper?
Massage	Uptight
Deep breathing	Holding breath
Good mother	No mother, bad mother
Good father	No father, bad father
Sensuality	Boring
A worthwhile activity	A waste of time
Good sexual memories	No sexual memories

For people who were profoundly deprived in childhood, you could make a similar list for extended eye contact.

After you have worked on the exercises in *Sex Smart* for a few months, go back and make another copy of the list of feelings about touch and circle the ones which apply. Compare the two lists.

Draw Your BodyMap

One of the best ways to discover how you feel about touch is to draw a BodyMap. Make two drawings of body outlines, one of the front of your body, and one of the back. Gather up three crayons or colored pencils, one blue, one red, and one green.

Now, imagine yourself in an affectionate, safe, and relaxed situation with someone you love romantically. Color in your two diagrams with the colored pencils or crayons, using this code:

RED = Do not ever touch me here under any circumstances.

BLUE = I may or may not want you to touch me here, depending on the situation and how I feel.

GREEN   =   I always like to be touched here.

Now, look at your BodyMap. If red or blue predominates, with very little green, it is likely that your ability to enjoy being sexual is severely hampered.

Which of the areas you colored in blue or red feel itchy or jumpy when they are touched? Take some time to think about what has happened in your family to create your own personal pattern of likes and dislikes for touch in each area of your body. Date your BodyMap for future reference, then read the following examples of what others have discovered.

> Dalia looked at her BodyMap and found that it had quite a lot of blue, very little green, and enormous areas of red under her arms, and on her chest and feet and legs. She recalled some bad experiences with touch that have left her feeling uneasy about turning her body over to another person.
>
> She commented, "From ages five to seven, my father tickled me against my will at bedtime 'til I had to call for my mother to stop him. Sometimes he stopped and sometimes he didn't. I liked the attention from my father because I loved him, but I got anxious and frustrated that he wouldn't let me control his behavior. It felt cruel and slightly sadistic. Even now, I find it hard to relax whenever my boyfriend, Bob, wants to hold me and cuddle."

> Brian's body map was almost entirely blue. He only had the tiniest portion of green, on the top of his head. Looking at his BodyMap, he commented, "My family was very tentative about touch. Come to think of it, they almost never touched me. The only place I ever got touched was some small pats on the top of my head. I guess this explains why I have the green there, and only there, and probably explains why I feel so awkward touching my wife, Debby."

Share Your BodyMap

If you have a partner, you can work with your partner using the Body-Maps. Share them and explain where all of the colors/feelings come from. Help each other to take blue areas and move them to a blue-green, and then to green. Always ask each other's permission to touch a particular area, and give each other feedback about how the touching feels. Never try to start out working on red areas, always on the blue ones. Redo your BodyMaps every three months or so, and compare them.

Look at Old Photographs

If you can't get many insights from drawing your BodyMap, there are other ways to recall your family's attitude about touch. Look at old photographs of you and your family at different ages. Who is touching whom, and in what ways? Are your parents touching? Are your parents touching the children? Do the patterns of touching change as the children get older?

Massage

Find a Massage Therapist

Go for a massage at least once a week over a long period of time. This can help you get in touch with your body and learn what types of touch you prefer. Be sure to communicate with your massage therapist to clarify your comfort level.

Take a Class Together

Massage is also a wonderful way for couples to support one another. By taking a massage class, you can learn how to use massage to help your partner with common ailments such as stiffness, soreness, or headaches caused by muscle tightness and stress. More important, you can learn about how to touch another lovingly, and how to be mindful of the intent that you put into your touch. And you can learn how to quiet yourself, center yourself, and listen to yourself and your partner.

Take a Class by Yourself

Sometimes, one member in a couple is so frustrated by the other partner's long-standing awkwardness with touching that bearing with that person through a couple's massage class would seem to create more anger. In that case, the problem would be best dealt with as a personal quest toward learning more about touch. In this case, each person can work on their issues about touch alone.

Practicing Touch

Use Clay

If your partner complains that your physical contact is too hard or too soft, you can work on learning touches of different strengths by using a malleable material that keeps its shape such as clay to rehearse. For example, if your touch feels too rough to your partner, first squeeze a ball of clay in your normal fashion. Leave that ball of clay as a model, looking at the depth of the marks which you made in it. Let your partner demonstrate the kind of touch that would please him or her. Practice squeezing other same-sized balls of clay, making progressively more gentle squeezes, until you are producing a squeeze that is pleasurable to your partner. Practice on clay until you get to the point where you are able to consistently gauge the strength of your touch, and can find a level that is pleasurable for your partner.

If You Do Not Have a Partner

Perhaps you have serious barriers with touch and love which have kept you isolated from other people, so that you do not have friends or a partner with whom to practice touching techniques. As remarkable as it may seem, even very long-standing and profound fears about giving and receiving touch can be altered, over time, if you are committed, financially and emotionally, to the process.

Other ways to explore touch:

- Join a class in dance or dance therapy.

- Get a pet or spend more time with a pet you already have.

- Join a gym in your neighborhood. You could even find a personal trainer.

After a year of trying one or more of these strategies, draw a new set of BodyMaps. Then take out your first set of BodyMaps and compare your progress.

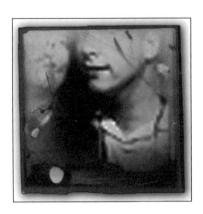

Chapter 2

The Foundation of Trust

The first real choice a human baby must make is whether to trust or mistrust other humans. The basic trust-versus-mistrust stage is the first building block upon which all later love relationships are formed.

—Dr. Ken Magid and Carole McKelvey, *High Risk: Children Without a Conscience*

♦ **Do you have trouble trusting others?**

♦ **Do you have trouble trusting your partner, even though you consciously realize that he/she is quite trustworthy?**

♦ **Do you have trouble relaxing in your body? Can you let deep feelings of relaxation in your body be a path into a sexual trance with a trusted person?**

As an infant, your waking world consisted of only two kinds of experiences—happiness and physical well-being, and unhappiness and pain. It was probably your parents who changed the negative state of the your babyhood existence—hunger pains or a dirty diaper—into one of satisfaction by feeding or changing or holding you. (If it was not your parents, you learned these early lessons about trust from whomever was your primary caretaker.)

If parents are extremely inconsistent in meeting the infant's needs over time, the infant will withdraw and become guarded emotionally. He won't expect parents to respond to his needs and won't reach out to be comforted or held. In turn, the parents may hold the baby less and less, further breaking down the baby's faith in the external world and others and the link between trust, empathy and affection, and physical relaxation.

As an adult, in order to even consider having friendships or falling in love, you need to start out with the assumption that if you have chosen your friends and loved ones well, that they will be there for you, to help and support you, if you need them. You must be able to trust another person when you are vulnerable, to know that it is safe to depend on another to care for you.

It is quite possible, however, that you haven't yet learned to trust. If you grew up in an alcoholic family, for example, you may have been the hero or heroine child; you may never have learned to ask to have any of your own needs met. Or, perhaps your parents were more negligent. If you suffered emotional and physical neglect or abuse which you haven't resolved, you will bring your old learned fears about pain, rejection, and abandonment into your current relationship, even if your partner is trustworthy. You will feel too vulnerable to allow yourself to let go and enjoy making love.

> *Sometimes I find that I have sex with a guy just to get him off my back, and then I'll refuse to see him again. I just don't trust men, and I don't want to take the chance of getting close. I'm confused about my inability to have faith in others. It seems to have many dimensions, but all of them are subtle. My parents didn't do anything terrible to us at all. They loved us. But there were dramatic financial ups and downs in our life that left me feeling unsafe. Maybe it comes from some of the awful experiences I had at school or at camp, where kids made fun of me. All I know is that I don't let anyone know what really makes me tick. And it comes out most dramatically in my fear of falling in love with a man.*
>
> —Mary, 34

Distrust

While good lessons about trust begin to be learned early, bad lessons about trust can be learned at any time during infancy, childhood, or adolescence. To the child, abandonment—real or threatened, physical or emotional—by the parents, is the equivalent of death. Unfortunately, if there were major problems with trust during your infancy, you won't be able to recall what taught you not to trust.

People who have learned to distrust in childhood can be irrationally hypervigilant in looking for signs of betrayal in their spouses or partners, even when partners have proven themselves to be generally trustworthy.

I think I can trace my difficulty with lack of desire and erection problems to ten years ago, when I had that back operation and I didn't feel that Sue was attentive enough to me. I guess it just stirred up all of those feelings of abandonment from childhood, like when I broke my leg riding my bike, and my father wouldn't take me to the hospital until the ball game was over on the TV. . . . I never really forgave her for that, and I never really talked to her about it, either.

—Vito, 55

Major breaches in trust during children's middle years and adolescence leave sexual scars, too. Children need to know that their parents care about them as they get older as well. Children see how much they are valued by their parents from the amount and quality of the time which is spent on them.

Having a parent present at performances or presentations is a clear sign to children that parents care. This is especially true when parents are clearly not there for their own pleasure or enjoyment. Child psychologist David Elkind (1981, 128) has commented, "Children view public presence of their parents as a visible symbol of caring and connectedness that is far more significant than any material support could ever be."

Adolescents continue to need the same kind of support they required when they were children, for instance, parents coming to a play or concert. They still need an affectionate hug or pat, even if they act as if they are too grown up for this kind of attention.

I was fighting a lot with my brother at this stage in life. One time I was in tears, and I remember running to my mother and asking her why my brother and I fought when I really loved him. She just looked tired and distracted, like she always did, and just said she didn't know, and for pity's sake, to leave her in peace.

—Bernice, 39

. . . I have come to realize how much time and energy I have spent, and still spend, in my life trying to manage all of the fear and anxiety I feel. I think I do not even acknowledge how much there is of it, most of the time, because I am so adept at managing most of it, and it is such a habit. I think how wonderful it would be if I didn't feel that the world was so threatening and I could use all that energy to do other things.

There are so many issues for me with sex, but what comes into my mind lately is that it just doesn't seem like a normal part of life for me. It seems separate somehow. Like when I am dealing with it, I am doing something apart from me. And it has become such a battleground for me. I have so many inner conflicts and fights about it. It sometimes just feels like big millstone around my neck, and when it's that bad, I can't even enjoy my husband touching me anymore, because even if it is nonsexual touching, it triggers all this uncertainty, and it takes me so much energy to conquer the uncertainty and the conflicts each time.

—Vonnie, 38

Facing issues of distrust learned in your family of origin is so painful that many people refuse to admit they exist, thereby perpetuating the "mystery" of the source of their sexual problems. Issues of distrust can lie at the root of almost every sexual dysfunction, including lack of desire, arousal difficulties, erectile difficulties, sexual pain, and problems with orgasm.

Beth's issues with trust contributed to her developing vaginismus, a kind of painful intercourse.

Beth met Bruce almost by accident, in college. Her neglectful childhood left her fearing other people, and she just had been beginning to make girlfriends in college. She had never even dated boys. But Beth and Bruce were on the same team for a whole semester in an advanced poetry class, and they got to know each other in a nonthreatening way, while reading Yeats and Dylan Thomas. That whole year, Bruce was going with Tina, a student at a college in a neighboring state, so he wasn't looking for a girlfriend.

The next year, Beth and Bruce were still on campus, but Bruce had broken up with Tina. He and Beth began going out. Bruce was a wonderful young man: funny, sensitive, gentle. They got quite serious, and made plans to marry.

Beth had never felt so close to anyone emotionally. She felt she probably could trust Bruce, because he really listened to her and he did what he said he would do. He liked her for all of the strengths which she, herself, knew she possessed. She began to have intercourse with him.

Initially, Beth enjoyed the sex, and was aroused (although not orgasmic). But the closer she got to Bruce, the more terrified Beth became of losing him. She had never experienced such emotional intimacy before, and it brought up in her an intense longing for connection that she never knew she had. She had always kept her wish for closeness in check, since she had experienced such deep disappointments in her family.

It was obvious to her that Bruce loved the sex, and she was beginning to believe that he actually loved her very much. There were times, though, that Bruce found it difficult to talk. Beth got scared at those times, scared that she would lose him, that he would go away. The feelings were too frightening to her. She didn't understand them exactly, and she couldn't talk to him about them. Beth began to use intercourse to keep Bruce close to her, at those times when he felt distant. She wasn't interested in or turned on by the sex, but the closeness with Bruce felt reassuring. The sex, however, was painful and Beth couldn't bring herself to tell Bruce that the sex hurt or how scared she felt when he got distant. Eventually, she developed vaginismus—a condition where the muscles at the beginning of the vagina began to have spasms, preventing entry. Beth had become so afraid of the pain of intercourse that she was tensing up.

Beth and Bruce got married, anyway. Beth got help with her sexual problem, and after a long period of reworking her painful childhood, overcame her issues of trust and was able to enjoy being sexual again.

Empathy

Good parents are empathic—they let themselves feel what their child is feeling, and then they respond to what the child needs. The more the child sees that the parents will respond to her needs, the more the child trusts that the expression of her needs is worth the energy expended to communicate. And so trust builds. Competent parenting creates children who are brave, creative, not afraid of risk. Children learn not to fear the potential hurts inherent in living, because they know that attachment and love can take many different kinds of hurt away.

They discover that if they fall and injure themselves physically, a parent's kiss can take away the pain. They find that if a friend hurts their feelings, their parents can give them a hug, use words to help them figure out what happened, and can reassure them that they are still good and lovable people.

Good parents actively engage in making the world safer for their children, constantly increasing the children's sense of trust. They change a child's teacher when they feel that that teacher is causing distress for no good reason, or they confront a bully's parents with the bully's actions.

Parents are major interpreters of feelings and of events for young children, since the children themselves are not good reporters of what has occurred. Good parents extend their own selves to spend a lot of attention on how their children are growing. They ask themselves, "What does this particular child need at this particular point?" in order to be the best parent they can be.

In general, adults who have been lucky enough to have had good enough parenting will be more optimistic about the odds of people coming through for them emotionally. Once they have picked a good-enough partner who is able to be empathic and soothe them, they re-evoke their childhood feelings and let themselves be soothed and calmed in the relationship. They don't feel chronically on guard, and they can go to other people for help when they have been hurt.

> Sally's father was a workaholic, and her mother did not have any capacity to be empathic or to follow through on promises which she made. Sally received almost no individualized attention in the family.
>
> Sally has no memories of time spent with her father. After work or on weekends, he went down to the basement to continue working or watch TV until it was time to go to sleep.
>
> Sally's mother would "forget" that she was supposed to pick her up at a Brownies meeting, and never show up. After Sally's father abandoned the family, Sally's mother was out partying the night before Sally was supposed to take her SAT exams in high school, and so her mother didn't get up in time to drive Sally to the exam.
>
> Sally's life experience left her with the following assumptions, assumptions that clearly have sexual corollaries:
>
> - If I get too close to someone I am not one hundred percent sure of, they will hurt and eventually reject me.
> - Most people are not what they seem, and they usually have ulterior motives for things.
> - It is better to do things on my own.
> - Deep down, I am too needy and expect too much out of most people, and once they find that out, they will reject me.
> - Other people don't want to hear my problems, really, and can't change things for me anyway.

Self-Soothing and Relaxation

When a baby is stressed, the parents are the ones to soothe him—their touch and soft voice can help the baby relax and feel pleasure again. Parents who are able to soothe their children raise children whose bodies are not tense or anxious, and the children tend to grow up to be able to self-soothe in healthy ways.

Are you able to close your eyes and experience deep relaxation? Can you imagine going to a safe place: floating on a lake on an inner tube, or lying on a blanket in a beautiful meadow, and closing your eyes and letting all the tension drain out of your body?

Many times, people from unreliable households experience trouble self-soothing and experiencing deep relaxation. Creating comfort for yourself in your own body may be the precursor to learning to be soothed by another.

Look again at your BodyMap. How much green do you have? Chronically anxious bodies have a difficult time feeling touch as pleasurable. Instead, touch feels too hard, too soft, or too ticklish.

If you constantly feel unsettled in your body, there may be no joy in giving up your body to another. It is too frightening to give up control, so while orgasm may be allowed, the sense of merging, or of turning into a pulsing mass of protoplasm is inhibited.

The foundation for your ability to really let go and feel the pleasure of sexual union with a loved partner rests upon your ability to trust and relax. Even if the process of confronting the past is painful, expanding your capacity to reach out and physically trust another person will pay great dividends.

Exercises

Increasing Relaxation in Your Body

Many people who are not able to experience the sense of deep relaxation and safety in their bodies aren't even aware that other people feel much more body safety. After all, each of us has only lived in the body we were born in.

If you grew up in a home where your parents taught you that life was dangerous, or if you grew up in a home which was neglectful or violent, you need to spend extra time and attention strengthening your ability to relax in your body.

Most relaxation techniques, books, and tapes assume that you are already have some skills: that you are able to tolerate physical relaxation, and that you can use the image of a "safe place" to go more deeply into relaxation.

If you find that intrusive thoughts of danger occur when your mind is blank, you need to slowly build up your tolerance for being quiet and focusing internally, minute by minute. Start by using a kitchen timer to start with just three or four minutes at a time. Then, try the following activities:

- Watch a video of a fire in a fireplace, or an ocean scene.

- Listen to an audio of rainshowers, the ocean, or New Age music.

- At the same time that you watch or listen, do deep, abdominal breathing.

If a frightening image intrudes, try to distract the thought by concentrating on your bodily sensations.

Create a SafePlace Image

If frightening images continually intrude, you will consciously have to work on creating a SafePlace. If your current life is, in actuality, safe, and if your current life-mates are trustworthy, try this exercise in cognitive restructuring. Fill in the blanks and cross out words so that this affirmation is true for you. Read it aloud. Then practice it once a day.

The household I grew up in was extremely _____ (e.g. chaotic, frightening, violent, unpredictable). It left me with me a lot of free-floating anxiety which I am learning to control and remove. Now I am safe_____ (alone; or with _____). I am secure. I can be calm. I don't have to be on guard, ready to _____ (watch that I'm not stabbed in the back, protect my sister, etc.).

It is safe for me to relax. It is good for my body and for my health for me to be calm. It is safe to be hugged and let myself float. No one will hurt me. I don't have to watch out for anyone else. _____ can take care of me. I have had times of peacefulness. In fact, the memory of _____ is a good image for a Safe-Place.

Create a Physical SafePlace

Another idea is to actually, physically, create a SafePlace in your house or apartment. Find a space (your bed, or a foam pad on the floor covered in a fabric you like), and surround it with art, music, or smells you like. Then you can practice going to that SafePlace when you get upset, do breathing exercises or refocus there.

Over time, hopefully you will be able to focus and relax for up to about ten minutes, and be able to create a SafePlace in your mind. Once you've accomplished that, you'll be ready for some techniques readily available in other books and tapes. What you will find is that your ability to relax just keeps getting better. After a few months, you'll realize that what you considered "relaxed" two months ago isn't as unwound as you can get now.

Trusting Others

Complete these sentences:

The scary thing about trusting people is _____

_____

_____

I would like to be able to trust more people, but I am afraid that _____

_____

_____

The times I felt most able to trust were when _____

_____

_____

The types of people I find it hardest to trust are _____

_____

_____

Where I Learned Distrust

List the three episodes in your life which made you feel the most abandoned or uncared for.

a. _____

b. _____

c. _____

These are the negative beliefs I gleaned from my lessons in distrust:

a. _____

b. _____

c. _____

Thinking of the most trustworthy people you know, challenge the general beliefs you have about people being untrustworthy with specific examples of times when friends, relatives, or co-workers behaved in a trustworthy way.

a. _____

b. _____

c. _____

What have been the general costs to you of holding on to your beliefs that it is not safe to trust anyone?

_____

_____

_____

After reading this chapter, which aspects of your sexuality do you believe are influenced by your feelings of distrust for other people?

_____

_____

_____

In the future in your relationships, how can you safely challenge your chronic fears about disappointment, betrayal, or abandonment?

_____

_____

_____

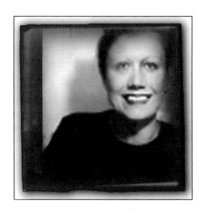

Chapter 3

Feeling Good About Your Body

Your body image is not the same as your physical body. It is the way you see it and experience your body, not necessarily how the world sees it—although how others experience your body can be very strongly influenced by the verbal and non-verbal messages you communicate about and through your body.

　　　　—Marcia Hutchinson, Ed.D., *Transforming Body Image*

A lifetime of experience goes into the creation of feelings about an individual's own body. . . .

　　　　—Lenore Tiefer, Ph.D., *Human Sexuality: Feelings and Function*

◆ Do you feel good about your body now?

◆ Did your parents touch your body in a loving, appropriate way while you were growing up?

◆ Do you think your parents felt good about your body when you were growing up?

◆ Do you think your parents felt good about their own bodies?

◆ As a child, were you put in charge of your body and all of its functions, at the appropriate time?

◆ Did you think your appearance was acceptable as an adolescent?

◆ Did your parents take major concerns you had with your looks seriously?

♦ **Do you think other people will find your body attractive?**

♦ **Do you have the ability to feel pleasure in your body?**

♦ **Do you feel good about your ability to feel pleasure in your body?**

Sexual feelings are body feelings. A sexual sensation can be a flush, a tingle, a warm surge, a rush. Whether or not you are open to these feelings and comfortable with them, experience them at all, or define them as pleasurable, depends on how you feel about your body.

Body image is a hefty part of self-esteem. It determines whether or not you feel good about yourself, whether you think others will be attracted to you, and whether or not you have the courage to approach the people to whom you are attracted. In short, your body image mediates your sexuality.

As you grew, your body image developed, contributing to feelings of sexual pride or sexual shame. How you have come to feel about your body as an adult was created by a myriad of influences. These include:

- how you were touched and held during your early years

- whether your parents continued to touch you affectionately and appropriately as you grew

- how well or poorly your body has performed for you in doing the necessary tasks and actions of living

- the continuing, often unasked for, assessments of your body by your parents, siblings, peers, and culture

To unravel and change your body image, you'll need to review all of these different influences.

While it is easy to criticize North American culture for the prevailing, mindless, focus on physical beauty, if you want to change your sexual self-esteem, you cannot afford to trivialize whatever assaults to your body image have occurred. You must work through them.

Being Sexy

Being sexy is, in large part, a state of mind. If you feel that you're sexy, you'll dress and act like you're sexy, and other people will respond to your sexiness.

Velda, a beautiful, heavy set heterosexual woman, was struggling with her own feelings about her weight and her lack of appeal to men. She was working on changing her sense of attractiveness. One morning, almost as an experiment, instead of wearing the loose-fitting, flowing clothes in which she usually dressed, she put on sexy clothes. Donning a short black skirt, black tights, high heels, and a V-neck top, she went out to run her errands one Saturday. Velda was amazed, several times that day, to find herself the recipient of appreciative looks from men.

Feelings of body freedom and sexiness are catching, too! One night, a group of friends went to a nightclub in the Boston area frequented by Russian émigrés. All of the women were easily fifty pounds and thirty years over the prevailing American "standard" for female beauty and erotic attractiveness. But no one had told them. They were wearing low-cut, sequined gowns (which many Americans would have said were "inappropriate" for "overweight" women), ecstatically happy in their own sense of their sexy bodies, entwined, and dancing up a storm, with their husbands and boyfriends. They made everyone watching them want to get up and dance, right then, and to go home and make love, later.

Since the mind is the primary sex organ, your negative feelings about your body constrain your bodily enjoyment. Sexual arousal is an individualized experience. Factors like the amount and distribution of the body hair you have, your height, your weight, or the size and shape of your breasts or penis do not determine how sexually responsive you are. But any negative feelings you have about your bodily characteristics put a damper on your ability to be uninhibited.

For instance, if you don't feel you are attractive, you might not allow yourself to get highly aroused sexually, because you won't like to imagine what you look like when you are "out of control."

Annika has an irrational fear of being too heavy. She has trouble enjoying sex unless she is a size six. She always wants to lose five pounds.

She would like to go to Weight Watchers to lose the "extra" weight, but they won't let her join. To join Weight Watchers, you must be at least five pounds over the lowest appropriate weight on the standardized height and weight table. Annika is petite—and so thin already she is almost off the chart.

Annika is a size eight now, and she still complains of being too heavy. "My stomach is flabby, and my butt is too big. I just can't enjoy sex at this weight. I'm too self-conscious."

A focus on real or imagined flaws will affect whether you are relaxed and can "go with the flow" in a sexual situation:

I feel self-conscious because my breasts are different sizes. I don't even like to turn sideways when I am with a man, sexually, because I think from that angle the defect is too noticeable.

—Genny, 34

I always make love with my clothes on at first. I wouldn't even consider taking off my pants before I had a full erection. My penis is so small when it isn't erect that I would never let a woman see me that way.

—Graham, 65

Body Image

Noted sexologist Leonore Tiefer, Ph.D., has emphasized the importance of early childhood experiences in forming body image. According to Tiefer (1979), in the first year, the infant gradually comes to recognize that he or she has a body, and that that body is separate from the world surrounding it. The infant also begins to form an emotional reaction to his own body, one which is very important to later sexuality. Mostly as a response to the baby-minder's response to the baby's body, the baby begins to feel very good or very bad about it.

Dr. Tiefer comments, "As the child continues to move around, feedback about the body continues to add to the developing body image. Is the toddler praised for efforts at coordination and grace, or is nothing ever good enough? Does the young child develop a feeling of being clean or dirty?" (pp. 36–37).

There is a huge variation in how American parents react to children's naïve freedom in talking about bodies and sexual parts. One three-year-old boy may look lovingly at his mother, as she gets out of the bathtub, and say "You're my breasty-girl" and get a motherly hug, while another kid might say, "Mommy, look at how big Tommy's wee-wee is," and get a slap.

Extremely chaste parents teach us that there is something not right about showing the body, talking about the body, or even acknowledging that we have a body—an inhibiting message that is difficult to break.

Some families are so emotionally cold and unaffectionate, or so focused on being cerebral or intellectual, that they act as if the child has no body. If you aren't taught to notice body sensations, you may just tune them out. If your parents didn't treat you as if your body was important, or valued, or even noticed, you won't be very attached to it, either.

> Tracy's parents were very undemonstrative during her childhood. There was no touching, no hugging, and no compliments. Tracy had no sense of her body as a source of pleasure, no sense of being physically attractive, and naturally, she wasn't able to enjoy being sexual with her husband. As she said, "John loves my body, and other men seem to be attracted to me, but I just can't seem to feel much of anything about my body."

Parents Who Hit

While growing up with an occasional spanking as punishment for a real misbehavior would not affect your body image, some families are out of control in the way they touch their children. Family violence, whether made up of child abuse or spousal abuse, sends a negative message about the body. Associations to touch are changed; touch no longer means safety and comfort, it means betrayal and danger. Nonsexual family violence makes such a huge impact on adult sexuality that it is dealt with in its own section of this book (see chapter 11).

Parents Who Tease and Criticize

When I was a teenager, I was really gawky. My father used to tease me and call me "eleven legs." I can't believe anyone would want to marry me. I always felt ugly. Too skinny, legs too skinny, nose too big, skin too pale.

—Alice, 28

As we grow, parents have an important and ongoing influence on our body image. Parents who tease, and those who are overly anxious or critical about their children's bodies have a destructive and long-lasting impact.

Sometimes parents have their own problems with body image, which they project onto their children:

> Chris is sensitive about his build and height. He reports that his father is obsessed and has been making an issue out of Chris's height for as long as Chris can remember.
>
> Chris's dad is enamored with sports and the "macho" ideal.

When Chris's mom was pregnant, Chris's dad had hoped for his own model boy: a strapping son. But first son Chris was always somewhat slight. After Chris, his sister was born, and then, four years later, another child, Bart, a son who was closer to Chris's father's ideal.

Chris turned out to be a responsible father and husband, and a steady wage-earner. Bart lived a life verging on criminality, flirting with drugs. Even so, throughout Chris's life, and even now, Chris's dad always comments on Bart's size and height: "Now your brother, Bart, you know how *tall* he is." But Chris's dad never comments on any of *Chris's* attributes.

Sandy thinks it is interesting that she feels so little pleasure having her breasts touched. Sandy's mother was a little overweight. As soon as Sandy began to develop, her mother told her to be careful not to gain weight, because it would show up in her breasts, and "Men hate big breasts." Now, every time Sandy gains a pound or two, she gets self-conscious about her body.

Other times, parents say cruel things comments which are never forgotten.

Rita has a port wine–colored birthmark on a portion of her chin. It's not very noticeable, but, despite her positive attributes (she's funny, pretty, has dark, curly hair and an attractive, lithe body), it has changed her whole life, and her self-concept. She became a set designer, rather than the career she aspired to as an actress, because of a cruel comment her father made when she was fourteen. Rita's father said to her, "With that mark on your face, no man will ever marry you."

Siblings Who Are Permitted to Tease

Siblings have an important role to play in the development of body image, as well, and part of parents' role is to prevent some of the "innocent teasing" that isn't so innocuous after all.

Thelma never felt cute after about age six. That's when she remembers her bothers starting to call her "big nose."

Josh has very full lips and feels hideously ugly. He can't imagine feeling any other way. Josh's two older brothers began teasing him about his lips when he was about seven or eight. They called him "potato lips" and "turd face." He felt helpless to get them to stop. His parents laughed his upset feelings off.

Now, eighteen, Josh can't understand why his girlfriend likes him. He discounts her sentiment that he is good-looking. His girlfriend adores kissing him, but Josh is so worried about the fleshiness of his lips that he really can't get into it.

Thelma and Josh's parents probably had no idea how much harm the "innocent teasing" caused to their childrens' body image and sense of sexual attractiveness. A lot of parents have heeded advice that siblings should "work out conflicts for themselves." It doesn't matter now, anyway, because as adults Thelma and Josh need to take responsibility for fixing the damage that was done to their sexuality. Even if their siblings apologized in adulthood, it wouldn't be sufficient to take away the hurt and the shame. Thelma and Josh now have critical voices inside themselves, voices which are activated when they are flirting, courting, or being sexual. Exercises at the end of this chapter should be helpful in combatting the internal critic and increasing sexual self-esteem and pleasure.

Parents Who Fail to Praise

Some parents, based on their ideas about the importance of pride and humility, believe that it is damaging to comment on a child's good looks. Since looks are "God given," these parents believe that it is wrong for the child to take pleasure in them.

Such dangers are overrated. None of us wants to produce a child who has a "swelled head" and who thinks that the only thing that matters about him or her is appearance, but the solution is not to refuse to say nice things about the child's physical attractiveness. Parents should balance their favorable comments between the child's physical attractiveness and the child's appealing character traits.

Greta only focuses on her perceived body flaws: her neck is too long, eyes too small, feet too big. When questioned about why she doesn't feel good about how she looks, she recalls her mother's voice: "Mother never felt it was okay to be proud of how her girls looked. She always said, 'My girls are attractive, not beautiful.'"

Greta grew up feeling it was not okay to feel pleased about her looks.

Parents who don't comment on a child's physical attractiveness are misguided. We all have what is called a reflected image. Our self-image comes partly from ourselves, and partly from the view of ourselves we see reflected back to us. If no one in the child's world ever comments on the child's cute body, beautiful eyes, beautiful hair, physical strength or gracefulness, or other charming physical attributes, the child grows up to feel invisible, or not very appealing.

Parents Who Neglect

Another way parents can hurt a child's body image is by not filling the role of caretaker of their child's physical body. Parents who do not address real problems affecting children's looks and physical functioning, whether out of ignorance or apathy, can damage their child's body image for life.

Sara, a woman in her forties, is one of several daughters from a lower middle class family in East Boston. Her father was emotionally cold and not very giving. Her mother drank. As an adult, she now knows that she has polycystic ovarian disease, which causes severe endocrinological problems.

Sara has been overweight since adolescence. She is very overweight now, with facial hair which needs to be shaved and, she says, hair on her belly. She feels incredibly ugly.

Sara's parents did not take her to a doctor when she did not get her menstrual period, as an adolescent.

Now, as an adult, she has finally received the medical care she needs. Even though some of her symptoms are now under control, Sara's sexuality has been damaged by feelings of self-disgust formed in adolescence. When she has a chance for a pleasant sexual experience, she can't let herself relax. She is too busy thinking about how revolting her body looks.

Additionally, parents need to teach their children about good physical hygiene. In *The Anatomy of Love* (1992), Dr. Helen Fisher describes how Americans, the Japanese, and many other groups find certain odors offensive. Children who aren't taught to properly wash their body and to brush their teeth can grow into adults who repel others simply on the basis of their smell.

Disabled Children

Children who have major physical disabilities or childhood illnesses may experience their body as so faulty, defective, or frustrating that life-long problems ensue. Or, some parents are so worried, or so taxed by the extra time and health-care demands that they tie the child too closely to them, hampering the child's wishes to socialize with peers. In the best case scenario, however, parents do everything in their power to enhance the child's developing sense of physical prowess, as well as to encourage the child's integration into the world of able-bodied and healthy kids.

Measuring Up

Children are acutely aware of their own body changes and constantly compare their own development with that of their friends, whether or not adults want to acknowledge such issues. Body image also plays a big role in how well or poorly children expect to be accepted by their peers, starting as early as age six, seven, or eight.

By early adolescence, children are very concerned with how they are measuring up to their peers. Cruel comments about other adolescents' bodies are common, among boys, among girls, and between boys and girls (see chapter 10).

Certain physical traits are very highly valued in American society, and not "measuring up" can lead to sexual problems. For boys, being tall and having a large penis are highly valued. For girls, the pressure is to be as thin and as beautiful as the models in the media.

> *I developed earlier than my peers in many ways. I got my period first, I grew breasts first, and I was fully a head taller than everyone else. School and sleep-away camp were both really tough. It was embarrassing to be the only person in my bunk who had to worry about sanitary napkins.*
>
> *In retrospect, maybe these girls were jealous, but they made my life hell. I always heard people whispering things about me. It made me very shy and awkward.*
>
> *Of course, now as an adult, everyone has caught up to me. I'm tall and thin, and that's really the cultural ideal, ironically. But somehow, when a guy indicates that he thinks I'm attractive, I don't believe it. I'm scared. I get this feeling that the situation is dangerous, that if I am a sucker and*

believe that he likes me or is attracted, that later on somehow I'll get attacked.

—Violet, 37

Height

Grant began sex therapy for premature ejaculation—he had always had a terrible time with it. The first time he actually "made out" with a girl in high school, he ejaculated inside his pants right away and had to pretend he hadn't.

Grant's problem persisted throughout adulthood. His marriage floundered partly because he wasn't able to hold off sexually; he got so excited when he entered his wife that he came immediately. Eventually he and his wife separated.

In therapy, Grant explored his body image and the possible connection between his height and his sexual dysfunction. Beginning in adolescence, he clearly didn't feel attractive to girls and historically, when he had sex, he seemed amazed that a woman actually would have him, and the physical excitement was often too much to control.

As a child, he had a lot of very tall friends. When he thought about instances in which he felt small, he thought of a few. In one, at about age seven, he and a friend were arguing about trucks. This friend was as big for his age as Grant was small for his. Johnnie, the other kid, got so mad at him that he just picked him up and hurled him into a sandbox, onto a bunch of trucks. Grant landed on a big backhoe truck and got bruised. Getting tossed through the air like that made him feel totally helpless.

There was another similar episode, later, where he got thrown around on a soccer field, ". . . as if I were a puff of air. . . . Again, I felt helpless."

He was only four feet eleven inches and one hundred and ten pounds entering high school. Grant looked very young; he didn't even get any muscular definition until he got to college. He wanted to play football, but he wasn't even tall enough to get on the team. All of these experiences left him with the belief, "My small size makes me inferior."

When Grant finally got into lifting weights, and had reached his full height (five feet seven inches), the girls began to take note. But this was after college. During college, he said, "I was just this pesky small kid buzzing around, trying to get everyone's attention."

Currently, actually, women are attracted to him. Grant is bright, ambitious, funny, and cute. But in his mind, he was stuck in the past.

Society's emphasis on height made Grant feel insecure in his adolescence. He didn't date much, partly because he was short, and adolescent girls actually did reject him. As this pattern continued, he became nervous around women. Even after girls began responding to him, his overwhelming anxiety abiout whether he would be seen as "good enough" and "manly enough" with women caused sexual problems. Thankfully, the standard exercises to control premature ejaculation are behavioral, and they are often helpful no matter what the underlying problem may be. Grant was able to cure his premature ejaculation, even though he continued to feel somewhat self-conscious about his height.

Dr. Alvin Poussaint, M.D., professor of Psychiatry at Harvard Medical School and senior associate at Judge Baker Children's Center, in an interview by Steinbaum (1994) noted that in the United States' pluralistic society, whole groups of shorter Mexican American and Asian American boys can feel insecure, when they compare their height to that of typical white boys.

Penis Size

Unfortunately, male concern with penis size may begin in early adolescence and continue through adulthood. Dr. June Reinisch, of the Kinsey Institute, reports that questions about penis size, shape, and appearance are, in fact, men's second most frequently asked question of the Institute. (Men's most commonly asked question is about getting and keeping erections.)

A national sex survey undertaken by *Mademoiselle* and *Details* magazines and reported on in *Details* (June 1993) asked a question about men's satisfaction with their penis size, and found a large amount of dissatisfaction among men with what the survey authors called their "magic wands." To the question, "Is your penis long enough?" many wished that their penis was either a little (39 percent) or much (6 percent) longer.

Some boys have unwarranted concerns about the size of their penis beginning when they are young children. If they cannot talk to adults and get reassurance (or medical treatment, in the very unlikely instance that something is physically amiss) their anxiety can lead to later sexual problems.

At age five or six, Solly decided his penis was too small. His obsession began when he began spending a month at a time at his relative's cabin in New Hampshire, and noticed that his penis was smaller than those of his same-aged cousins, Brad and Gregg. Showering, he looked over and was disturbed to see how far out his cousins' penises protruded. He later saw his uncle's penis and became further concerned.

Solly was alienated from his harsh father and too shy to talk to his mother, so he kept his worries to himself. The fears built and built. He felt ugly, unattractive, and sexually undesirable. As an adolescent, he was afraid to ask girls out, for fear that they would make fun of him. When he finally began having intercourse, he had problems with premature ejaculation, which made him feel even worse about himself.

Even though he is married now, he still feels inadequate. He has retreated from his anxiety into a fantasy world. He is obsessed with sexual thoughts all of the time, and secretly undresses (in his mind) all of the women he sees.

Boys' locker room competitions about penis size are probably the biggest source of anxiety about adequacy of penis size.

I always dread communal showers. I am very ashamed of my small penis. I remember, when I was in junior high, I decided to go on a bicycle outing in Colorado, sponsored by the YMCA. It was a rugged ride, through the Rockies, up steep mountain passes. We went long distances, and slept outside and at youth hostels. At the hostels, we had to take group showers.

One horrible evening, as we were taking group showers, one of the other participants, also a teenager, looked over at my penis, and said, 'Geez, Bob, you'll never get up this next mountain with that thing!' I never forgot it.

—Bob, 38

For men, the concerns with height and penis size are elevated by open verbal competition and hostile remarks, on the playing field or in the locker room. Because the adult men of today have been socialized to be secretive about their vulnerable feelings, particularly about sexuality, each of the many adult men whose self-image was wounded in adolescence believes that only *he* has had this harrowing experience.

Pornographic movies also leave some boys and men feeling insecure. They forget that the actors are hired precisely because their penis size is extraordinary, and that the movies are shot from an angle that exaggerates the size of the actor's penis.

Sometimes, girls and women's sexual ignorance and cruel comments leave a boy or a man with tremendous anxiety about his body image. Women who falsely believe, "the bigger the man, the bigger the penis," occasionally seduce tall men into bed.

I have seen several tall men in my practice for body-imagery problems caused by encounters with exploitative and uneducated women who lured them into bed out of sheer sexual curiosity—and then could not conceal their disappointment.

> One girl told Jeff, "I thought that you would be really big, you know, but actually, you're smaller than some of the other men I have known who are shorter than you."
>
> Jeff found it hard to get her comment out of his mind. He said, "I'd like to run away somewhere. I feel inadequate, useless."
>
> The time that Jeff actually had a serious, committed relationship with a young woman, they had a wonderful sexual relationship. She thought Jeff was perfect. But when he broke up with her, he found that his anxiety about what other girls might say to him when they became sexual made it really difficult to begin dating again.

Breast Size

For girls, who develop physically before boys, there are concerns with being at the "right" level of development at the right time—getting your period neither noticeably before nor after your peers, and development of breasts of the right size at the right time.

> *As I walked down the hall, the boys would call out, "Hey, are those things REAL??" These breasts have been a pain all my life. I can't get clothes to fit. I still feel scared when I walk by a group of men. And I have to say, I really don't feel much pleasure when my breasts are touched.*
>
> —Anna, 32

Being Thin

In case you hadn't noticed, the media images of female beauty are getting thinner and thinner (Steinbaum 1994). The body measurements of *Playboy* centerfolds has fallen so much that the average *Playboy* centerfold is now 15 percent less than normal weight, which also happens to be the clinical definition of anorexia. From 1959 to 1979, the weight of contestants in the Miss America Pageant shrunk substantially, and it has stayed down.

So the "ideal" American woman now is one with an eating disorder! And, with the constant pressure of these body types on television screens, on billboards, and in magazines and newspapers, we probably see more "perfect" people in a day than normal ones.

American girls have started dieting earlier and earlier. A 1994 study by Jennifer Read, M.Ed. (Department of Psychiatry, Beth Israel Hospital, Boston) presented to the American Psychological Association Annual Meeting found that a mere 30 percent of eighth grade girls were content with the size and shape of their bodies (Steinbaum 1994, 21).

Being Pretty

Even when the problem isn't weight, despite feminism, the pressure on girls to be "pretty enough" is formidable. Many girls carry into adult sexual encounters the feelings of rejection they received during adolescence.

After years of nagging by my family, I finally have focused a lot of energy on looking good . . . But there is a down side. . . . Men seem to be attracted to me now, but I just can't trust it. . . . I thought the highlighted hair, the contact lenses, the makeup, and the working out would fix it, but it just can't. . . . I can't relax. I feel intimidated, and I expect rejection.

Sometimes I just hate men. . . . Inside the new, attractive me, lies the sixteen-year-old who didn't get invited to the junior prom, and the seventeen-year-old who had to import her own prom escort, a distant cousin from another state. . . . If I get close to a man and want to become sexual, I actually find myself picturing taking off my clothes and him laughing at my stretch marks. I don't think there are any exterior changes I could make which would make me REALLY feel good enough, pretty enough, inside.

—Estelle, 26

The "rule" that women be thin and pretty is so resolute that some men, evidently, feel that it is their right to harass women who don't fit it. Over the years, several of my overweight female clients have reported their repeated experiences with verbal attacks by strangers while in public places. For instance, while on a subway or in a crowd, a perfect stranger will approach them, saying something like, "I just had to tell you how completely disgusting-looking (or ugly, or fat, or hideous) you are." Needless to say, these women are very frightened of social situations, and would never dream of approaching a person to whom they were attracted.

In a survey of women readers quoted in *Family Circle* magazine (February 1, 1994) money was rated the number-one stress, "weight problems" ranked as number two, and "body image" as a separate category came in at number six.

Every era has its "look," especially for women. In America during the 1920s, for instance, the idealized shape of a "flapper" included small breasts, and many women bound their breasts tightly to achieve that look. In the 1940s, a more voluptuous look was popular so for the next years, women wore bras that were constructed to push the breasts up and out.

Soon after, surgical techniques for breast augmentation became more available. Now the current fashionable shape seems to be one that appears quite infrequently in nature: a lean, athletic body with well-rounded breasts. Currently, an estimated 72,000 women yearly choose to surgically increase their breasts.

Further, at least in the United States, *youthful* beauty is equated with sexuality. Don't believe for a minute that to *feel* sexy in your body, you must look like the idealized beauty standard currently popular.

Cultural Standards

Body image is based in part on the culture in which you were raised. Some religious cultures distrust bodily pleasures. They forbid even nonsexual activities—such as dancing—which might evoke sensual delight. Growing up in a subculture like this, it's hard to feel really comfortable with your own body, not because it isn't sufficiently beautiful to qualify as being sexual, but because it is alive, and thus, is *too sexual*.

> *When I was growing up, in the Pentecostal Church, I played the organ. I got a lot of attention for being a good musician. Everyone praised me for being so good, such a good Christian. At the same time, I developed early, and began to get in touch with sexual desires (to masturbate) when I was*

eight or nine. But these desires were forbidden, and I wanted to be a good Christian. I was literally at war with my body.

Even now, as an adult in a marriage, I still feel uneasy when I get swept up in sexual feelings. Sometimes, right in the middle of being passionate, I want to put on the brakes. I feel bad. I have to consciously step in and tell myself, "Tim, these feelings are okay. These feelings are natural." My wife, who wasn't raised in the same kind of church, doesn't understand. She is incredibly frustrated with me.

—Tim, 49

Looking Good

Most of us are average looking. When average-looking people walk down the street, no one turns around to look at them, one way or the other. Average-looking people have some nice features, and some not-so-great features, but overall, their looks are clearly "acceptable." People who have exceptionally attractive appearances are not statistically the norm—nor are the equally small number of people who have unusually poor looks, for a variety of reasons—genetics, a medical condition, bad luck, fire or accident, and so forth. This is a serious problem, sexually, that no one talks about much. What should you do if you really do have unusually bad looks?

There is no doubt: having terrible looks will make it harder to attract friends and lovers throughout life. As Dr. Rita Freeman says (1988), "looks-ism" is rampant in our country. Freeman documents study after study showing that good-looking people get special treatment, and poor-looking people are discriminated against, whether it be in romance or when trying to get a mortgage. For average-looking people, the trick to managing body image is to accentuate the positive in your looks. As one of my friends said to herself in the mirror, "Well, you don't look like Michelle Pfeiffer, but for me, you look pretty good."

If you are especially plain or unusually bad-looking, you still deserve love and eroticism—everyone does—and you might need some special tips to get up the nerve and energy to get what you want. One problem you may have faced over your life is that no one, including your family, was willing to discuss the fact that you were, in fact, being rejected by others solely on the basis of your looks. The denial of your reality may have left you feeling more isolated.

Children and adolescents are really amazingly cruel. You may have suffered from such viciousness when you were younger so that you now freeze up in sexual situations.

> *. . . When he touches me, even though I know he loves me, I just freeze up. I can't feel anything in my body. I think I mostly feel fear. All those years of getting taunted by those kids, hearing those voices:"fatty, fatty, two-by-four, can't fit your body through the door."*
>
> —Martha, 26

At the most extreme, your experiences in childhood and adolescence may have been so dreadful that you developed social phobia: you are so frightened by rejection or humiliation that you avoid contact with others as much as possible. If so, you have to tackle your social phobia first.

If you reacted in a less strong way and don't have to tackle full-fledged social phobia, what should you do? Well, you have to do the best you can at playing the hand that you're dealt. While your family and close friends may have been denying the reality that people reject you based on your looks, and that that creates difficulties in attracting a partner, you yourself may be overemphasizing the hopelessness of the task.

You have to examine the way you are thinking about things and assess whether you are overemphasizing the negative. Consider these truths: While it is true that, in general, you are being discriminated against for your looks, it is *also* true that just as there have always been looks-snobs, there have always been people who look *below* the surface at people's inner beauty. So, cultivate your other personal potentials. Once you work on your self-esteem and strengths as a person, then force yourself to be social, to go out in the world and meet other people.

In addition, never underestimate the power of conversation skills— often what starts out as a friendly attraction, *can* become sexual attraction. Remember the brain *is* the largest sex organ. Fortunately, with such modern conveniences as the Internet, the possibilities of attracting other people on the basis of your other interests and traits are becoming increasingly strong.

Be the Best You Can Be

Growing up in American culture, each and every one of us has been bombarded with unrealistic images of what it takes to be "sexy." There is major pressure to try to become a perfect, thin, young, sexy, beautiful woman, or an equally gorgeous, tall, muscular man with an enormous penis (capable of instantaneous, consecutive erections).

It becomes clear, then, just how important having had a supportive family environment can be to developing a healthy body image—a contentment in having your own, normal-looking face and body. Our family experience can provide the antidote to these ridiculous stereotypes of what kind of body it takes to be lovable, and what kind of body can feel sensual and sexual pleasure.

If we're lucky, families provide the touch that makes us know, from the skin inward, that we deserve love, and that our bodies are sources of pleasure. Families can make us aware that we are our bodies, and that that is good. They can give us compliments about our physical strength, abilities, and appeal at different ages.

At best, families can provide an enviroment in which we can get shelter from the cruel comments of others. An adolescent who can talk to his or her parents about other kids' cruel barbs can get the empathy, inner strength, and comfort needed to weather the years until adulthood. And families can provide the emotional and financial resources to change or repair our bodies, when genetic flaws cause us to be so uncomfortable living in our God-given bodies that our feelings of social confidence are diminished.

As adults, of course, each of us is in charge of how well we do with the bodies we have. Use the resources at the end of this book to get started on doing the best you can with what you have been given.

Exercises

Identify Bad Messages

Close your eyes and imagine a sexual encounter with a loved person. Remembering that the mind is the most important sexual organ, identify any negative messages that you give yourself about your body, or any harsh comments that you believe your partner might have about your body.

Trace the source of your bad feelings by making a list of the first, or worst, time you had issues with any part of your body

This Problem Began with:

	My own feelings	My family environment	My peers	Culture
Feeling I am unattractive in general				
Hair				
Height				
Weight				
Breasts				
Penis				
Other aspect of general appearance				
Feelings about touching genitals				
_____ (other)				
_____ (other)				
_____ (other)				

Assess Reasonable Goals

Look at the previous list and mark with a "C" (for "change") those items about your body, *or your feelings about your body*, that you could healthfully change, and an "A"(for "accept") next to those things you cannot. For instance, while your height is probably not changeable, your feelings about your height are. (If you are insecure enough about some changeable aspect of your body such as your teeth, it is okay for you to reparent yourself and spend some money on correcting the problem.)

Then write here your ideas for ways you might accept the "A"s on your list.

_____

_____

_____

Remembering that you don't have to be physically perfect to feel sexual pleasure or to continue to grow sexually, pick two areas marked "C" and state what your goals are for changing.

1. _____

2. _____

Rework the Past

List here significant critical incidents from your past where others have wounded your body image. (Use more paper if necessary.)

_____

_____

_____

Then write letters to yourself, your peers, parents, siblings, or media moguls saying what positive message about your body you wish you had received.

_____

_____

_____

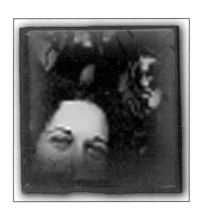

Chapter 4

What You Learned
About Gender

*The processes whereby our maleness and femaleness are determined,
and the manner in which they influence our behavior, sexual and
otherwise, are highly complex.*

—Robet Crooks and Karla Baur, *Our Sexuality*

♦ **Are you happy being the gender that you are?
Why or why not?**

♦ **What did you learn about being your gender in your family?**

♦ **Do you buy your family's definition of how you should be
and act?**

♦ **Who were your role models for your gender identity?**

♦ **Has your gender identity been affected by your sexual orientation?**

Gender

Not much is simple about the concept of gender. You were born a particular
sex (that is, male or female), but you weren't born a particular gender. This
is because there is a difference between the terms "gender" and "sex." Our

"sex" refers to our biological femaleness or maleness. Actually, there are two different parts to our biological sex. First there is our genetic sex, which is determined by our chromosomes (a normal male has two sex chromosomes, an X and a Y; a normal female has two X chromosomes and no Y chromosomes). The second aspect of our sex is our anatomical sex: the obvious difference between having male or female sexual organs.

How secure you feel in your gender is an important ingredient in your comfort with being sexual. Think about it: Gender is the very first thing we notice about another person! In order to be comfortable being sexual, you need to feel good about the sex you were born (male or female).

Gender Identity

The term "gender identity" refers to our own, individual and subjective sense that "I am a male" or "I am a female"—with all that that gender means for you. Each of us constructs our sense of gender differently, depending on the era in which we live, the society in which we live, and our family. Being comfortable with your gender identity is an important part of your sexuality: without the formation of a gender identity, none of us has a framework within which to have a romantic relationship with another person.

Sex therapists are fond of saying, "Your biological sex is between your legs and your gender identity is between your ears!" Gender identity development results from a complex interplay of biological and social learning factors. The question of which—biology or learning—plays the larger role is still being hotly debated by researchers. *Sex Smart* will address what you learned in your family about gender.

> *I wonder sometimes whether my mother's weird version of femininity has affected my security in my gender. She was in some ways appallingly passive, and yet she was very giving emotionally. As a kid, I vowed never to be that passive, and I'm proud of my accomplishments in law. But I'm also not as devoted to my husband or kids as my mom was. Sometimes I worry that I'm not feminine enough. When I gain weight and my husband isn't as interested in me sexually, I totally withdraw, and sex comes to a complete halt.*
>
> —Ruth, 58

Gender Role

Based on the biological sex of a newborn infant, parents immediately begin socializing their baby to be a proper little boy or girl, inducting them into their gender role or sex role: the attitudes and behaviors which are considered normal and appropriate in a specific culture (and during an individual era) for people of a particular sex. The terms "masculine" and "feminine" often come up as descriptions of what a society in general thinks should go with the sexual differences: "feminine" describes attributes that we think should go with femaleness, and "masculine" describes qualities which men should possess—and these cultural definitions perpetuate what children are taught about gender. In American culture, little boys are swung around in the air, and called "tough" and "strong" and "big boy" and "tiger." Little girl babies are protected and called "little sweetie." But definitions of proper "feminine" and "masculine" vary with each culture. Anthropologists such as Margaret Mead (1963) studied cultures such as Tchambuli society in New Guinea, where patterns of masculine and feminine behavior are opposite of our American norms.

You learned about gender from what your parents told you, and by watching each of your parents and how they constructed their gender role, and how your parents interacted. If you didn't like what you saw in the model your father or mother set out for you, sexual issues may result. You also learned lessons about gender from your peers and from school.

My parents were very protective. Each time I had (and was proud of) an adventurous or challenging experience like playing with older kids, exploring the neighborhood woods or field, my mother would turn out to be panicked for my safety and punish me by restricting my movements even more.

—Vicki, 60

It's a good thing that I had my best friend's father as a model: He was a scientist, and a quiet guy, but very kind and loving. I could never measure up to my father's version of manhood—some beefcake of a guy who only thought about sports and sex.

—Hal, 33

Margaret's mother found her father kissing another woman when Meg was five. The mother began telling Meg that "All men will cheat when given a chance." Meg has trouble trusting men.

What About Sexual Orientation?

It is important to realize that gender identity is separate from sexual orientation. Your sexual orientation may be heterosexual (attraction to the other sex), homosexual (attraction to your same sex), or bisexual (attraction to both sexes). Despite stereotypes and the fact that a small proportion of homosexual men and women dress and act in opposition to their biological sex, most homosexuals are happy with their gender (Crooks and Baur 1993). In fact, a study by Storms (1980) measured general gender-role attributes and found no significant difference in characteristics of masculinity and femininity among homosexual, bisexual, and heterosexual male and female college students.

> *Sometimes I think about how distant I felt from my Dad, and whether that has any relationship to my homosexuality. I'm not sure they're related. To me, my sexual orientation seems more like a biological kind of thing, something that existed in me from the very beginning. Having a cruel father didn't help things, but I don't think I'd be straight if he had been different.*
>
> —Sam, 48

However, there is no guarantee that your gender identity or ideas about your proper gender role will be consistent with your biological sex. Transsexuals, for example, have profound conflicts between their sense of gender identity and their biological sex.

Others of you may simply not buy into societally defined gender roles—for example, that women are less interested in being sexual than men are; that men are active and women passive; or that men are more knowledgeable than women in matters of human sexuality. So although your sense of your gender goes along with your anatomy, you are not willing to follow the "rules" (or myths) that society has set out for how to be a proper boy or girl, or man or woman.

> *Oedipal stuff wasn't important. I never could identify with my mother. I didn't want to be a housewife and a mother, and I never was in love with my father. I identified with my older sister, who was independent, and my first 'in love' experience was with a male teacher who was nothing like my father.*
>
> —Bettina, 40

My mother was really into this submissive woman kind of model. She was forever telling me things like, "Don't wear your heart on your sleeve." The message I got was that as a girl, I had to let the boys initiate everything. *I don't think that I could have been like that even if I wanted to. The funny thing is, I think that the men I have dated have really liked the fact that I ask for what I want.*

—Olivia, 30

I find that I am really blocked, now at twenty-three, by being a virgin. Men just aren't supposed to have gotten this far in life without having intercourse and I am just terrified at this point of trying to actually have sex with a girl. She'll be able to tell that I'm a virgin, and I'm afraid I'll die of embarrassment. At this rate, I'll be a virgin when I'm forty!!

—Bryant, 23

Feedback from a parent that you aren't "masculine" or "feminine" enough to please them the way you naturally are will undoubtedly damage your self-esteem and your sexual self-esteem. Your parents' rejection of your gender role identity, and/or sexual orientation may make it seem threatening to get into a sexual relationship with another person in adolescence and adulthood.

Sexual Behavior: How Your "Sex" Affects Your Sex

Your beliefs about what is appropriate behavior for your gender affects many aspects of your sexual experience. Children who learned to feel inadequate as the gender they are, as adults, feel sexual fear, shame, and embarrassment. In some cases, obvious sexual dysfunctions are created.

When Trudy was a girl, her mother dressed her like a boy, and cut her hair in a bowl-cut. She gave Trudy books, but not frilly clothes, barrettes, or jewelry. She dressed her in boy's red plaid shirts and strangers assumed that Trudy was a boy.

When she grew taller, at age ten, her father further undercut her sense of femininity by calling her "mommy long-legs" and teasing her that if she stood sideways, she would be invisible. In addition, Trudy's parents were very prudish about sexual matters.

When Trudy wanted to know what a tampon was, she was repri-manded. Sexual matters were not discussed at all, and when Trudy got her period, there was no discussion about anatomy, bi-ology, relationships, or sexuality. Her mother simply gave her a sanitary belt and told her to stay away from boys and focus on her studies.

Trudy later developed vaginismus—and after entering sex therapy had to reconstruct her sense of her own femininity before she could get control of her vagina back. Trudy's sexual fears, inse-curity, and genital pain were directly determined by the way in which her parents failed in the task of her gender socialization, even while they may have meant well.

Donatella, a high-powered lawyer, began sex therapy complain-ing of being frozen sexually, of having no sexual desire whatso-ever. While she had succeeded in breaking her culture's gender roles by becoming a prosperous and well-respected professional, she still felt inferior as a woman. Although she married, she had never enjoyed sex with her husband.

In therapy, as an exercise, she was asked to rent a few movies which she thought might have appealing and intense sexy (though not necessarily sex) scenes. She came in the next week after having viewed two movies and reported that she had a mixed reaction to both of them. Part of her was turned on, but another part was turned off to the fact that "Sexuality in those movies was con-trolled by the man. He was being selfish and it was his desires that were being acted upon. In one of them, the man spent ninety percent of his energy trying to get sex, *not* trying to get to know the woman."

In beginning to explore Donatella's feelings, she voiced a lot of other attitudes about men and about sexuality: "I hate it. I hate it the way men just use women sexually. They just view all women as sexual objects, there to please them.

"You should see the guys in the law office ogle the secretaries. They don't even care what the woman is like as a person—to them she is just a sexual object. It's disgusting."

From there, Donatella went on to talk about her resentments toward her husband, an attorney much older than she.

"He has all the power. What gets done is what is at the top of *his* priority list. If he wants something, I go along with it. If the kids or I want something, and he didn't think it up so it's not on his list, he won't go along with it."

As we tried to distill her belief system, it boiled down to these tenets:

- Men have all the power.
- Men make all the decisions.
- Men use women sexually.

Donatella put her sexuality in the same categories: Sexuality was all for her husband's needs. If he wanted to be sexual, he bothered her by touching her. When she objected, he told her that he wanted her to feel good. But her feeling was that "It's all about your needs. You want to make me feel good so you can have sex. But I don't want it."

Donatella was furious: "Women are really submissive, in every relationship I see. Here I killed myself, with loans and studying, to get through law school, and I'm still submissive!"

It seemed to me that these attitudes probably came from earlier days, from before her marriage. What had she seen in her family of origin that made being a woman look so oppressive to her?

Donatella remembered, back from when she was ten or eleven or twelve, that her mother was "always aggravated that my father got to have fun and go out with the guys. She stayed home all day with all those kids, and worked her fingers to the bones cooking and cleaning, making all the meals, laundry, cleaning up. Even in the evenings, she always had babies to take care of. She never stopped, she didn't even take time off to talk to a girlfriend or make herself a cup of coffee.

"And my father was not romantic at all and didn't act appreciative. And when my father did decide that they would go out in the evening occasionally, he'd just tell her that afternoon, 'We're going out tonight,' and leave her scurrying around trying to get all her work done, and trying to fix her hands and her nails, because they were all ruined. She never had any chance to prepare for it or to get ready."

At that point, Donatella said, "I told myself that I never wanted to get married." And Donatella withdrew from men. She didn't date. She threw herself into her studies, to prove to herself that she could be a woman and have power, too. However, in her thirties, she decided that she wanted children, and she did marry.

But Donatella's alienation from her gender role made it feel as if she couldn't "submit" to sex and still feel good about herself. Even if she liked sex, if her husband liked it more, and since all men wanted was sex, than she couldn't let herself like it. Donatella's feelings about her gender caused problems with sexual desire and arousal. Her unwillingness to identify with her mother made it difficult for her to come to terms with her sexuality as a woman.

If you have grown up in a family where you are ashamed of the behavior of your parent of the same sex, but you admire the parent of the opposite sex, you may find it easier to identify with the feelings of your opposite-sex parent, leading to sexual problems.

Gary came into sex therapy for treatment of his erectile dysfunction. He was caught in between two girlfriends, one an old girlfriend from college who really loved him but whom he no longer loved, and a second one, a woman he had met at a computer conference and had exchanged email with, who was much more sophisticated and wild.

As we talked, his conflict became clear. He was terrified of hurting his old girlfriend, with whom he was trying to break up, so he couldn't perform with his new girlfriend.

Gary's father had abandoned Gary's mother when Gary was thirteen, to go off with another woman. Gary was old enough when it happened to have very clear memories of how badly his mother was devastated emotionally. She had cried for months, and he had done everything he could to comfort her. He had taken over as the man of the house. His father had left them badly off financially, too, and Gary had worked hard to bring in more money. He had total contempt for his father, who he rarely saw.

What caused Gary's erectile difficulties? Gender identity issues! When Gary hurt his old girlfriend, leaving her to go off with a new love, he awakened his unpleasant gender identification with his masculine role model, his father. Gary had never put his feelings about his father's behavior into words before. He hadn't realized how negative he felt about being a "man like my father." He needed to verbalize his feelings about his father, and also to redefine masculinity for himself. When he came up with a more caring, sensitive version of masculinity, Gary got his ability to have erections back.

So, as you can see, your feelings about gender are an important component of how comfortable you feel about being sexual with a loved person. Your relationship to your parents, your feelings about how they defined their gender roles, their feedback to you about how well you fulfilled their gender role expectations of you, and your feelings about their relationship to each other have all influenced your sexuality.

EXERCISES

The three major words I could use to describe my mother's relationship to my father are:

1. _____

2. _____

3. _____

The three major words I could use to describe my father's relationship to my mother are:

1. _____

2. _____

3. _____

Fill in the blanks:

I assume that men will _____

_____

I assume that women will _____

_____

Spend a day turning these expectations on their head. How does the world change if you treat the opposite sex the opposite way?

_____

_____

_____

How have the messages you learned about gender in your family affected your expression of your sexuality?

_____

_____

_____

On a scale of 1–10, with 1 being extremely happy and 10 being extremely unhappy, how happy are you with the gender you are?

_____

_____

_____

Why or why not?

_____

_____

_____

In what ways have societal definitions of gender-appropriate sexual roles affected your sexuality negatively? Complete each sentence about society, then complete each sentence about yourself, listing more empowering or less constricting gender role definition.

1. Society says I should be / do _____

_____

_____

I give myself permission to be / do _____

_____

_____

2. Society says I should be / do _____

_____

_____

I give myself permission to be / do _____

_____

_____

3. Society says I should be / do _____

_____

_____

I give myself permission to be / do _____

_____

_____

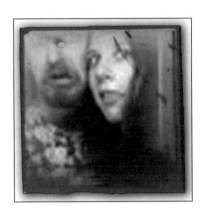

Chapter 5

Feeling Good About Yourself

*[To succeed, romantic love] asks a reasonably good level of self-esteem.
If we enjoy healthy self-esteem—if we feel competent, lovable, deserving
of happiness—we are very likely to choose a mate who will reflect and
support our self-concept. If we feel inadequate, unlovable, undeserving
of happiness, again we are likely to become involved with a person who
will confirm our deepest vision of ourselves.*

> —Nathaniel Branden, "A Vision of Romantic Love," in
> Robert J. Steinberg and Michael Barnes' *The Psychology
> of Love*

- ◆ **Do you love yourself?**

- ◆ **When you look in the mirror, do you feel excited by your own
  potential?**

- ◆ **Do you love and accept your physical body and take good care
  of it?**

- ◆ **Do you feel that you deserve to get good things?**

- ◆ **Can you figure out what you want and need?**

- ◆ **Can you ask for what you want in social situations?**

- ◆ **Can you ask for what you want in sexual situations?**

- ◆ **Do you feel comfortable in a relationship where someone loves
  you and values you for your good qualities?**

Self-Esteem

Self-esteem is *the* major ingredient in feeling good about yourself, which in turn determines a lot about your ability to be emotionally intimate and sexual with others. Satisfying intimacy within a relationship *begins* with self-love: a genuine interest, concern, and respect for yourself. As a small child, your self-confidence and self-respect was either nurtured or subverted by the adults in your life, and depended on whether or not you were respected, loved, valued, and encouraged to trust yourself. But since those early years, your self-esteem also has been influenced by the choices and decisions you, yourself, have made.

Self-esteem has two parts, according to Nathaniel Branden, author of *How to Raise Your Self-Esteem* (1987): a feeling of personal competence and a feeling of personal worth. It reflects your implicit judgment of your ability to cope with the challenges of your life, and to master them, and of your right to be happy—to respect and stand up for your interests and needs.

According to McKay and Fanning's book *Self-Esteem* (1992), studies of young children show clearly that parents' style of child-rearing during the first three or four years determines the basis of the child's self-esteem. After that, most studies of older children, adolescents, and adults do not find it easy to delineate the primary influences of high or low self-esteem and their effects.

Any time a man seems to be falling in love with me, I find myself pushing him away. When I think of undressing, honestly, I get nauseous—that's how afraid of the inevitable rejection I am. I just can't stand the pain of him finding out how empty I am inside. I can't figure out what it is that he sees in me.

—Sue, 29

At this point, I'm just so anxious about my erections that I don't ever feel safe sexually with Tricia anymore. Each time we try to make love, I just feel like such a failure. I know how much she likes the feeling of me in her. She should be able to count on me to be able to do this for her. I feel like a failure, big time. I can't get these negative voices out of my head. It's getting to the point where I don't even want to start anything, for fear that I won't be able to finish it.

—Kevin, 45

If you were lucky, you had normal self-esteem by the age of three or four. A child who feels secure in her own worth and identity within the family is able to reach out, to get close to others, first in friendships with peers—in playgroups, nursery school, kindergarten, and primary school. Later, in adolescence and young adulthood, if you had good self-esteem you used these same skills you learned in being friends with other children, and went on to form love-based, mutually satisfying sexual relationships.

On the other hand, not having self-esteem leads to making poor choices in friendships and love objects. In part, this comes from a lack of knowledge about what a loving relationship feels like. Partly a person stays in an unhealthy relationship because she doesn't feel she can ever do better—and this only perpetuates a downward spiral of less and less self-esteem.

> Alana grew up in a family with critical, distant parents. Her feelings of inadequacy, caused partly by learning disorders, led her to feel like a nobody at school. Her parents did not pay much attention to her school problems, so that Alana never did well at academics. She also felt aloof from her family.
>
> At fifteen, Alana "solved" her problem of low self-esteem by getting involved with Troy, a boy six years older than she. Alana's parents were so uninvolved with her that they didn't stop her from going out with a boy so much her senior.
>
> Although she didn't particularly feel valued by Troy, he had a car, and Alana felt that being seen with him would give her status at school. Alana felt more like one of the "cool kids." Unfortunately, Troy didn't really love Alana. He cultivated a highly sexual, somewhat exploitative relationship with her. This left her with even worse feelings of worthlessness than she had had before she met him. In addition, as an adult, she had to struggle with sexual problems caused by the ruthless way in which Troy disregarded her feelings during sex.

If you don't feel good about yourself, it may not occur to you that you are a good enough person to have a kind partner—this may lead to choosing a lover who is overly critical, addicted to substances, abusive, etc. Furthermore, you may be confused over whether or not your partner is really treating you badly, whether or not the relationship problem is your fault, and whether or not you are simply "getting what you deserve." Subsequently, leaving even a poor relationship is difficult, because you desperately want the small positive benefits you get from the current relationship (i.e., living in a nice house, or a sense of "belonging" that is better than one you had as a child) and don't really believe that you are good enough to do better. Staying stuck in the poor relationship further damages your self-esteem because it seems to prove your lack of worth to others and to you—thus perpetuating your declining self-esteem. Low self-esteem may also cause you to be more vulnerable to sexual trauma in adolescence and reinforce the negative effects you may have suffered as the result of violence in your family (be sure to read chapters 10 and 11).

> Sam grew up in a chaotic family, with a mother who was hospitalized several times during his early years, and a father who went out to work but had nothing left over for the children when he came home.
>
> There was no sense of order in the house, and none of the children felt valued. Many times, there wasn't enough money, and the family lived in housing where there were not enough beds for everyone. Sometimes Sam's father would drink, too, and collapse on the couch (which was Sam's "bed") so that Sam had trouble sleeping. The children weren't kind to each other, either. Sam's older sister would awaken him in the early morning, while he slept on the couch, by putting on a bright light so that she could iron her clothes. Sam literally didn't feel that he had a place in the world. He felt he wasn't worth much.
>
> He was very frightened of relationships with other kids and later was not comfortable with girls. He didn't date much, because he was too frightened of rejection. Finally, in his midtwenties, he was "chosen" by a woman who wanted to marry him. After several years of marriage, it became clear that the woman was a chronic gambler and was putting them further and further into debt. Nevertheless, Sam was too frightened of feeling abandoned and alone again, and he stayed with his wife.

If you grew up with a parent who was continually critical, it is likely that you have developed an internalized critical monologue, often unconscious and automatic, which can cripple your self-esteem to such a degree that it makes it difficult and painful to get through the times in a relationship when a partner is angry or faultfinding of you.

> David grew up in a home in which his father was continually criticizing his every move—he had struggled for years with his feelings of low self-esteem. A homosexual man in his early thirties, he had been struggling to find a stable partner for some years. When he finally met Frank, David knew that he wanted to get serious.

They became very close to each other emotionally and had a healthy, loving emotional and sexual bond. After a year, they moved in together.

But once Frank and David made the commitment to each other, David began to feel insecure, and to have sexual problems. They entered sex therapy, to figure out what the cause might be.

When Frank and David began living together, small conflicts inevitably arose: for example, Frank was a neat-nik, and David was not used to being tidy. When Frank began to fault David for being a slob, David felt his old anger from childhood welling up. But he was too frightened of Frank leaving him, of losing Frank's love, to actually talk about his feelings. Instead, David tended to withdraw. Instead of focusing on simply changing the small behaviors that bothered Frank, or having the confidence that with enough talking they could work out whatever the problem was, he froze. David became progressively more obsessed with the idea that he had ruined Frank's life, that he couldn't do anything right, and that Frank would leave him. When they were making love, these feelings and thoughts created enough anxiety and self-consciousness to interfere with his erections.

As it turns out, David's inability to deal with conflict in an intimate relationship was related to David's critical father and David's lack of self-esteem. In therapy, Dave learned to challenge his father's perfectionism and reassure himself with several correcting thoughts: that he and Frank were a team and Frank loved him, that Frank was *not* Dave's father, and that Dave *could* please Frank.

Kevin grew up in a rather repressive home, with parents who administered a lot of discipline and very little love. His father, who worked as a physicist, was gone a lot of the time. Even when his father was home, he wasn't present emotionally. His mother seemed upset to be trapped at home with the children, and seemed to take very little pleasure in Kevin and his siblings. Nevertheless, she was the favorite parent, since at times she showed some concern and love.

Kevins' mom's standards for his schoolwork were very high, and he was forever disappointing her. He really longed for some closeness and for her love, but eventually, he simply put these feelings away. He became a very meticulous adolescent, perfectionistic and self-critical.

Kevin was too much of a nerd to date much in high school, but when he got to college, he began to date. He fell in love with an engineering student, Tricia. All of the longing for love he had held back from his childhood came out in a gush, and Kevin was startled by the strength of his feelings of yearning and love.

Things went very well in the beginning of the relationship, and Kevin and Tricia got married. Both Kevin and Tricia worked, and life was good, as was their sexual relationship. However, after they had children, Tricia decided to stay home for a few years. After a while, she became resentful at Kevin for not participating with the children.

Kevin was devastated at Tricia's criticism. It awakened old feelings from his childhood, and he began to have erectile difficulties. The problem got worse and worse, with Kevin withdrawing totally from Tricia.

When they finally went to sex therapy together, Kevin finally realized that his constant feelings of self-criticism during sex made his performance anxiety even worse. Things got better as both partners understood their role in the problem. Tricia understood, now, that her criticism had awakened long-smoldering feelings of being abandoned, and she became much more complimentary and understanding. Kevin began to consciously talk back to his internal critic and deal with his performance anxiety by focusing on his own sexual pleasure and by reminding himself of the many different pleasures he could give to Tricia, even if he had occasional erectile difficulties.

It's Not Too Late

You might be asking yourself what you can do now about your problems with self-esteem, if things have gone badly for you thus far. The answer lies in identifying and manipulating your own internal negative *schemas* about the present. A schema is a belief system you use to organize your understanding of life and to help you make decisions. A negative schema is usually based on injurious experiences you actually had in your past.

Some examples of negative schemas (Korn 1997) would be the following:

- All people will abuse me, hurt me, or manipulate me.

- There is no meaning or justice in the world.

- I will eventually be abandoned.

- I am not capable of functioning independently in life.

- I am powerless.

- I must be in control of everyone and everything around me.

- I am bad, disgusting, unlovable, defective, evil.

- I'm a freak, an alien.

As you look at these schemas, perhaps you might recognize one you hold. I hope that you will notice that if you make current life choices as a result of any of these schemas, you are guaranteed not to get what you want.

For example, look at the first schema: "All people will abuse me, hurt me, or manipulate me." Regardless of the abusiveness of your past, of course you will want a future life filled with people who will love you and treat you well. However, if you follow this negative schema in your current life, you will most likely either avoid relationships altogether or fall into a negative one, since that is all that you think is possible.

In almost all cases, no matter how dire your childhood, if you challenge your negative schemas, and force yourself to take responsibility for making more optimistic choices among all of the possibilities the future holds, life will improve.

There are numerous small things that you can do to raise your sense of competence and general self-esteem. And each of these "little" things will then influence your sense of sexual self-esteem. Each small step can be very frightening to do, but just pushing through the fear itself, and making more optimistic choices, is very empowering. Self-esteem is critical to healthy sexuality.

> Lucy grew up in an atmosphere of total emotional neglect and developed into a fearful person. She felt frail in her own body, frightened of danger, and afraid that others would reject her. She was lucky enough to be married to a wonderful man, but she didn't feel secure enough to relax during sex, or to ask for what she wanted in their sexual interludes. She couldn't have orgasms.
>
> In therapy, it became clear that her whole life was constrained by the dread she felt. She confessed that in the summer, she wouldn't even wear shorts on a hot day, because she was so frightened that people might look at her body, or might say something upsetting to her. To challenge this fear, we decided that Lucy

should start taking walks in her neighborhood—a very frightening idea. Lucy pushed herself to take these walks, in graduated steps—first brief walks wearing pants and long-sleeved tops, and finally taking longer walks wearing shorts and a short-sleeved blouse. It was a liberating process to challenge her fears. To her surprise, no one said anything awful to her, and the neighbors were friendly and called out to her. As she felt more powerful and competent in the world, and more comfortable in her body, asking for what she needed, sexually and socially, came more naturally. As Lucy could ask for the specific kinds of touches she liked from her husband, she became orgasmic.

The relationship between sexuality and self-esteem is circular. Being sexual *per se* is a poor way to deal with a deficit in self-esteem. Sexuality cannot be safe and healthy if you are being sexual with someone who exploits you or doesn't consistently care about you.

Developing good self-esteem sets the stage for good relationships with trustworthy people. Lucy's example, literally overcoming the results of a neglectful, lonely childhood and low self-esteem step-by-step, is a good metaphor for you if you need to recover your self-esteem.

The exercises which follow will help you realistically assess the choices you have made which have enhanced or dampened your self-esteem so far. If you spend time on the exercises in this chapter (and utilize the resources for this chapter—see page 255), you will be more likely to wait until you have a relationship in which there is emotional intimacy and commitment. At that point, being sexually intimate may well further enhance your self-esteem.

Exercises

Assess Your Self-Esteem

Write down the three things you like best about yourself:

1. _____

2. _____

3. _____

Imagine that you want to make contact with someone you don't know, but to whom you are attracted. Imagine that you have to "sell" yourself to that person. Write a 20-second commercial for yourself.

_____

_____

_____

Oftentimes, low self-esteem leads to poor choices in friendships and lovers. If you think you've made such choices, fill in the following chart.

Person I chose who was bad for me	Reason I chose him/ her	Bad belief I gained as a result	Correcting Belief About Myself
_____	_____	_____	_____
_____	_____	_____	_____
_____	_____	_____	_____

If you have made poor choices in your relationships in the past, describe here the kind of sexual partner (or friend, if you haven't become sexual yet) you want and deserve.

_____

_____

_____

Low self-esteem sometimes makes it difficult to ask for what you want sexually, even in a healthy relationship. If you have been secretive about your sexual wishes in a healthy relationship, compose a list of those wishes here. Try to arrange the wishes in order, starting with the ones which might be the easiest to ask for, and ending with the ones which would be the most threatening to ask for. Then write in today's date and a target date by which time you will ask for each of these wishes.

	Today's Date	**Target Date**
Wish 1		
Wish 2		
Wish 3		
Wish 4		

Assess Your Sexual Perfectionism

No one has the perfect body, and no one is the perfect lover. If your sexual self-confidence is marred by the rigid, perfectionistic demands you make on yourself, document them here. First list the demand you make of yourself that makes it threatening for you to participate in a sensual or sexual situation with a loved person. Next, write yourself a soothing statement which you can use the next time you judge yourself so harshly. Using this statement will help you overcome your criticism and move forward into the desired sexual situation.

1. Criticism _____

   Retort or Correcting Thought _____

2. Criticism _____

   Retort or Correcting Thought _____

3. Criticism _____

   Retort or Correcting Thought _____

Low self-esteem often leads to perfectionism, which can interfere with your ability to relax and focus inward on your own sexual pleasure. If you are now aware of that pattern, list your distracting, perfectionistic thoughts, and next to each, write a focusing or breathing image which will help your body experience pleasure by focusing on an activity or a part of your body you like. (For instance, "I will ask to be touched on my thighs and focus on how erotic that feels.")

Perfectionistic Thought or Belief During Sex Which Inhibits Pleasure	**Competing Way to Focus on Pleasure**
_____	_____
_____	_____
_____	_____
_____	_____

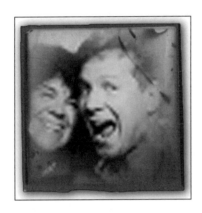

Chapter 6

The Dynamics of Power

The measure of a man is what he does with power.

—Pittacus

♦ **How controlling were your parents, in general?**

♦ **Could you express your upset or angry feelings appropriately to them? Were you allowed to disagree with them?**

♦ **Can you express your upset or angry feelings to other adults now?**

♦ **Do you find yourself concerned with issues of control and vulnerability when it comes to sexual relationships?**

Parental Authority

The way in which your family handled power is key in your experience of love and your expression of sexuality. If authority was handled well by your parents, and they were empathic caretakers, you have grown up associating being in a relationship with love, comfort, and getting your needs met. The issue of dominance probably causes few major conflicts or stumbling blocks for you in your sexual and intimate relationships.

If, on the other hand, your parents greatly abused their authority over you, you have learned to link emotional intimacy with power struggle. If this has been your experience, you may find you have trouble integrating love and sexuality. An enormous variety of sexual dysfunctions and problems—including sexual aversion, low sexual desire, difficulty relaxing during sex, difficulty becoming excited or coming to orgasm, and sexual compulsions and addictions—can be related to a lack of parental empathy combined with authoritarian dominance.

If your parents were quite controlling but also loving and not abusive, you may fall somewhere between these two extremes: it is quite possible that your sexual relationships will be marked by some ambivalence or by power struggles.

> *All of my issues of power come out in my relationship with Jeremy, even though he is the most loving person I know. But I just fight him whenever he wants his own way, and that happens in sex, too.*
>
> *This therapy is exhausting. I'm in a state of grief. I don't want to admit this stuff we're talking about. Mom and Dad's crazy rules. My resistance. I don't want to replay the scenes of fear, listening to them talking about me through the vents of the house, hearing my father's steps on the stairs . . . my terror of getting beaten. Getting a black eye for something as dumb as taking my brother's baseball cap.*
>
> —Shelley, 36

Parents of infants, while they may be overwhelmed by the many tasks at hand, are quite clearly in charge: infants are tiny, not yet articulate verbally, and their only desires are to have their physical and emotional needs met. A power struggle at this age is futile and highly unnecessary.

But soon the child becomes a toddler, and begins to say, "No!" to what the parents want and makes demands herself. She ambles about, carrying things, and the soap winds up in the fishtank, the spoon in the toilet, and the house becomes a shambles. This stage (also known as "The Terrible Twos") is where the control battle begins between parent and child.

Mother to two-and-a-half year old:	"Sally, Don't climb up that high chair. It will fall over on top of you and hurt you."
Two-and-a-half -year-old to mother in response:	"No. Shut up. I hate you!"

By the time children are four, they are making it clear that they have their own personalities and their own wishes. Parents do more or less well with their childrens' increasing independence. A father who used to flirt and call his little girl "my little kitten," suddenly may withdraw love and approval as that little girl tells him she doesn't want to bring him his slippers when he comes home from work. Another parent may take pleasure in watching what appeared to be a very docile child become intent on leading his or her own pursuits.

Of course, at this age, the parents are still in control. Consider the small child who is throwing a tantrum and refusing to leave the swimming pool on a very hot day. He can be hoisted up, simply and easily, by the adult and be carried to the car, all the while screaming his head off, arms flailing.

If the parents are kind and loving, and wield their power justly, there is no problem for the child's developing sexuality. But some parents are not well equipped psychologically for the task of parenting. They are depleted by all of the child's demands, and they are much more prone to use control and violence than they are to give love and tenderness. If the parents are not empathic and loving, and they act sadistically, the issue of power and control can impact the child's general personality and sexuality in a very destructive way.

In order to comprehend how the issue of power and control can be woven into a child's personality and sexuality, you must be willing to think of the parents as the object of the child's greatest love. In actuality, the parents are both the child's dearest love and the source of the child's worst frustration. Besides their advantage of physical strength and size, they have the emotional power to say no or to gratify the child's desires.

If parents are kind, empathic and giving, the house is run like a kind of benevolent kingdom, where the parents rule but are humanitarian heads of state who try to do what is best for the populace and take their subjects' wishes into consideration. If the parents are dominating, the household feels like a cruel dictatorship.

Of course, the parental-child power dynamic changes as children grow up. As children reach about eight years of age, they become more independent, more adept at expressing their thoughts and wishes, and more able to use their behavior to rebel against what they feel are unjust rules. They can run away, they can talk back, they can refuse to comply by flaunting family rules. By adolescence, children are large enough physically, and independent enough, to mutiny against parents who wield their power without justice or love. In general, though, children who grow up in cruel and authoritarian families express their feelings of rebellion by self-injurious behavior—depression, not doing well in school, withdrawing from social contact. As will be described in the chapter on adolescence (chapter 10), teenagers are even more adept at self-harm, including using drugs, sex, fighting, or driving too fast as distractions and / or to express rebellion and independence.

What was the control pattern in your family of origin? If you could express frustration overtly to your parents, within reasonable limits, that was healthy. Many parents are sophisticated enough to know that it is normal for their child to tell them they are the meanest mother, or father, in the world.

But a little boy who hears his small girlfriend call her mother a "witch" with no punishment may go home and try it out in his family and may get a slap, or his mouth washed out with soap. If you came from that kind of family, and you were tyrannized by your parents, your sexuality may have been inhibited or associated subconsciously with aggression or control.

> Greg grew up the oldest child in a loving but controlling home. His mother, a psychiatrist, was vibrant and fun, but also quite intrusive and demanding. His father, an orthopedic surgeon, had high hopes for his son. Greg was given a lot of financial advantages, including being able to ski in Europe several times a year, private day school, and the financial backing to take many kinds of private lessons.
>
> Since childhood, Greg had always dreamed of being an artist; however, from about the age of eight on, his mother and father made it absolutely clear to Greg that they expected him to be a lawyer or a physician. Ironically, his family was so well off that the financial instabilities of a career in the fine arts really would not have been a problem.
>
> Because Greg was so bright in English, science, and math, his parents assumed he liked these subjects and could not understand why he couldn't just go to law school or medical school. He fought them through his teens, but eventually Greg capitulated and went to law school. He became a reluctant, unhappy lawyer.
>
> Greg met Harry when they were in their early thirties. They were extremely attracted to each other and formed a monogamous relationship after about a year. They had a lot in common, and in most areas they did not argue or compete. However, Greg's issues with power came out in their sexual relationship.
>
> Harry's sexual drive was much higher than Greg's was and the discrepancy set off all of Greg's feelings about submission. He simply was not going to do what he had had to before—give in! He wouldn't consider negotiating, or taking turns about whose sexual preferences should win out. He out-and-out refused to discuss

their desire discrepancy, let alone go see a sex therapist. Eventually, Harry felt so hurt and so discounted that he left. Greg's old feelings of losing the power battle with his parents made him so unable to negotiate that he eventually lost an important love relationship.

Linking Love and Sexuality

Children Are Innately Sexual

While most of us don't think of youngsters as being sexual in any way, they are indeed. They just aren't sexual in exactly the same way that adults are sexual.

Children can have wonderful, romantic feelings toward their parents, particularly the parent of the opposite sex. And of course, children experience great sensual pleasure in their bodies, from being hugged, rubbed, or getting their back scratched. So children with empathic and responsible parents, particularly parents who touch them lovingly and appropriately, develop a sense that people they love can be a source of deep emotional and sensual pleasure.

And as anyone who has caught a small child masturbating knows, children's bodies can have sexual sensations of buzzing and throbbing the same way that adult bodies do. But unless a child is in a sexually abusive environment, exposed to inappropriate information and experiences (where an adult is using the child to fulfill adult sexual needs), children's "sexual" fantasies have nothing to do with explicitly adult activities like sexual kissing, petting, oral sex, or intercourse.

Early Fantasies: Sex and Control

Children's sexual fantasies are much more vague. Often, they can be fantasies of control. Many children have enjoyed playing eroticized games of control with each other.

One little boy ran around, at age five, rubbing his penis on little girls, and scaring them, "because it feels good, and it's fun"? Girls may be lacking penises, but they have their own sexualized control fantasies.

Sarah remembers playing a game of "Mean Queen" with her two sisters when they were about five or six. The person who was the Mean Queen got to give out orders. One order which appeared frequently in the games was the Mean Queen telling her commoners to wipe her rear end!

Masturbation in Childhood and Adolescence

Children and adolescents often use their newfound sexual pleasure derived from masturbation as part of their control fantasies as well. As power struggles may be going on between parent and child, the child definitely has control over his fantasies, and, in masturbation, control over his own body.

According to sexual expert Leonore Tiefer, Ph.D., in all cultures studied, more boys than girls masturbate. This probably has to do with boys' access to the penis, or maybe with the experience that boys have in touching their penis as they learn to urinate. (Interestingly, boy monkeys masturbate more than girl monkeys, and they don't touch their penis to urinate, so the gender differences in rates of masturbation must have to do with more than just physical access to the genitals.)

Masturbation may also be used as a means of self-comfort and escapism. For more about masturbation and adolescence, read chapters 9 and 10.

Depending on the family environment in which you were raised—how you were taught about power and control, whether or not you were allowed to question authority—early patterns of control fantasies (involving masturbation or not) can set the tone of your adult sexual life.

Tom came into sex therapy with his wife, Jackie. She complained that she hated their sexual relationship, that he was unable to be loving or tender, and that he treated her like a sex object. He didn't touch her body tenderly—he just grabbed for her breasts. In addition, he was very attached to having Jackie go along with certain staged scripts in order for them to have sex, which alienated her. Jackie wanted their lovemaking to be full of tender moments. Tom said he just wasn't put together that way. Tenderness just didn't turn him on.

Tom loved his wife a lot and could not understand what was upsetting her. He knew that he had always had a high sex drive, that he was very attracted to Jackie, and that he wanted her to be available sexually. She complained that sex didn't occur in an atmosphere of romance, but that instead it had a pornographic, controlling tone to it. Tom just couldn't see what the problem was.

He grew up in a family with a loving mother but a physically and emotionally abusive father. Tom's father hit him, called him names, and made him feel worthless. Tom knew his mother loved him, but she didn't protect him.

As a young boy, Tom discovered the pleasures of masturbation. He learned that when his dad made him feel rotten, he could lose himself in the pleasures of masturbation. He began a pattern of masturbating to a script where sexy girls made him aroused. The excitement and orgasm temporarily distracted him and took his emotional pain away. He continued to masturbate for pleasure and escape from his youth until the present.

Because of his loving relationship with his mother, he was able to love his wife and children, and to be a good husband and father in many ways—but his rigid sexual pattern created a major problem in his love relationship with his wife, who felt hurt at the lack of tenderness. With much work, he was able, eventually, to be soft and sexual occasionally, but his primary route to arousal continued to be highly scripted, pornographic fantasies of *Playboy*-type women.

In unsympathetic and controlling families, the child can grow into adulthood associating relationships with nothing but control: fearing any kind of closeness to another person; sensitive to control themes everywhere; or concerned about the submission implied in a sexual relationship.

It's funny, in my dreams, I am doing a lot of screaming at my mother, and it reminds me of how antagonistic we were to each other. I guess it started when I hit puberty. I just couldn't stand being around her or hearing that commanding tone in her voice and I would fight with her and argue and yell about being asked to do even simple things, like clear the table or do the dishes, or take my feet off the sofa. Anything.

It was this battle for control, and I felt like she was trying to control me and I would have rather died than do anything she asked, no matter how small. There were even a couple of times when she tried to physically make me do stuff, but I was strong enough to make that impossible for her to do.

Later on in college I had a roommate. She was very similar to my mother in the sense that I found out very quickly that she had certain ideas about what her roommate should be like, and I did not fit her idea . . . She couldn't leave me alone. She kept saying things and doing things to try to get me to be what she wanted. I couldn't get along with her at all. I grew to hate her. I can't stand being around people who are controlling. Feeling accepted for who I am has really became a very important thing to me in life.

—Jenny, 40

Discipline

Dominance and Submission

Playing with issues of dominance and submission in the context of adult, sexual relationships can be fun, as long as each of the partners has a choice about whether or not to engage in the activities. Unfortunately, children of controlling parents—to whatever degree—do not have a choice. The end result being that they can't have fun in relationships, because they are too afraid. They can't role-play with issues of power and control. They can't let power issues be fluid, shifting back and forth. Children of domineering parents are locked into a single role, so frightened by power that as adults they feel they must *always* be in control—or must *always* submit.

> Rob, an only child, grew up with a rather cold mother and no father. His mother may have meant well; she certainly meant no ill. However, she lacked empathy, and wasn't affectionate. She had very high standards for a child, insisting that Rob do well in school and also be very helpful around the house. Rob felt quite dependent on her emotionally and otherwise, since they lived in an isolated area and he had no siblings.
>
> Occasionally, she gave him beatings where he had to lie across her lap while she hit him across his buttocks with a hairbrush. Even though Rob was clothed during the beatings, he remembers experiencing them as mildly erotic, particularly since he didn't get held and cuddled all that much. His sexuality developed around themes of masochism: women with whips, women treating him like a slave, or women treating him like an animal. He could not become aroused in a situation of tenderness or emotional closeness.

Sexual games of dominance and submission for adults can be a variation, a way to spice up sexual life. But when the only variety of sexual interaction which feels good, and the only means of sexual arousal, revolves around strict, fixed roles of dominance and submission, this implies that something was terribly amiss in the power dynamic in the family.

In Rob's situation, he flipped his feeling of being victimized around in his mind. His erotic desires remained intact, but only in a situation where power roles were well defined, and he could be in a scripted game where he could choose to be controlled. In George's case (see below), his unconscious link between power and sexuality growing up in a controlling family caused a complete absence of sexual desire.

George was brought into sex therapy by his second wife, Sima. He had no sexual desire and was struggling with erection problems. "Sex is just a job to me," he said. In fact, he reported, he had never been much interested in sex.

Sima was hurt and upset by his attitude because she truly loved him and used sexual relations for comfort, for connection and relaxation. George always avoided her sexual overtures and never seemed interested.

George came from a background of overwhelming control, physical abuse, and emotional neglect. Besides being given no physical nurturance, George was frequently shoved, slapped, and spanked to the point of bruising.

In addition, there was emotional abuse. George was called names, embarrassed, and was allowed no expression of his own needs. His father bellowed, "How dare you ask for _____," if he ever requested to get his own way. In his mental imagery of childhood, being hurt and losing control figured prominently.

George's family governed his every move, even into adolescence. The parents owned a successful shoe repair store, and from the time he was six or seven, he was expected to work in the store before and after school, with his silent, critical, angry father. He was not allowed to take time to have normal relationships with peers: no softball games, Boy Scouts, or any other activity.

Whatever sexual urges he did have terrified him. He certainly did not want to be controlling or aggressive with another human being. He barely had an opportunity to date, because he wasn't allowed to have any free time. He couldn't bring anyone home. In adolescence, he parked with girls a few times, but never went beyond kissing.

As soon as he could, he left his harsh family and went into the army. When his army mates found out that he was still a virgin, they took him to Pigalle, a red-light district near Paris, and bullied him into having sex with a prostitute. He was terrified and the experience upset him deeply.

As George reexamined his history, he began to see a connection between power, control, and his repressed sexuality. His current problem seemed to be that he was angry at Sima for the way she was spending money. Unexpressed anger is often connected to lack of sexual desire.

Sima knew that she and George were having conflicts, but she could tolerate her feelings of disappointment at George. She could fight with him over control issues, yet still feel her sentiments of love for him and continue to be sexually interested in him.

But George could not stand to think of himself as an angry man. In fact, he was actually afraid of his irate feelings, so he repressed them. He could not stand to see himself as the kind of seething person his father was. He could not express his anger nor ask for what he wanted. He just shut Sima out and felt himself not attracted to her.

Most importantly, George just didn't think of himself as a sexual person. (It seemed that he had never discovered masturbation.) George's lifelong distaste for sexual expression was related to his abusive childhood. His associations to touch were violence and fear, not pleasure. Once when George was asleep on the couch, Sima looked down at him and felt such love that she came up and kissed him gently on the cheek. George jumped up, startled! He felt that Sima was trying to control him sexually as well as financially, and continued to feel vulnerable.

George had learned to be fearful of aggression and any wish to control. He could not imagine a constructive way of changing his relationship with Sima. In the process of simply surviving the brutality of his life, he shut his feelings off, including his sexuality, and could not integrate power and love.

Some children from homes like George's recognize the abuse and break away in adolescence (whether escape is healthy or not). They seek solace elsewhere, in other friends, by using drugs, or, like Tom, in the temporary relief of sexual arousal and orgasm. George was overwhelmed by the oppression. In turning off his feelings about the abuse, he also turned off his ability to love, to deal with conflict, and to feel sexual desire.

Sexual Criminals

There is a direct link between families who abuse power and the creation of sexual criminals. Parents who lack empathy covertly reinforce the child's aggressive behaviors toward others. In a study of forty-three adolescent or sibling incest perpetrators, Pierce and Pierce (1990, 102) commented, "It appears that juvenile offenders frequently reside in families where they receive minimal warmth and care."

These authors found that 63 percent of the abusers had been physically abused in their family themselves. In several other studies of incestuous fathers, common themes from their childhoods included overwhelming physical abuse, abandonment, powerlessness, maternal seduction, and paternal rejection.

Of course, only a tiny percentage of people who grew up in abusive homes wind up becoming sexual predators. But, in all of these examples, you can see the range of sexual adaptations to different family power profiles.

If you grew up in an angry, controlling family yourself, it takes a lot of courage to look at your past. Most people who grew up in a violent home minimize the problem. Even George, who we met in this chapter, doesn't describe himself as having come from an abusive background!

And as George's case illustrates, growing up with abuse affects people differently. In George's case, it destroyed his sexual desire. In Tom's case, he had strong sexual desire, but his fantasies tended to link sexuality and control. He was able to love, but couldn't integrate tender sexuality with love. Sexual addiction, which will be addressed in chapter 10, is another common outcome of growing up in a family in which power was misused.

A Sense of Owning Yourself

Think again about the relationship between power and sexuality. What lessons have you learned in your family?

Parents who controlled you all the time were abusing their power—this shouldn't have occurred—and as a result you have learned bad lessons about how horribly power can be misused by loved or trusted people. You must now intentionally *un*learn them in order to have a healthy, equal sexual relationship with another person.

If power was abused in your family, many sexual problems may have resulted. You may not have a sexual drive at all, like George. You might have problems with intimacy because of unrelenting power and control issues, like Greg or Jenny. You may have become sexually compulsive, using sex not to connect with another human being, but instead to soothe yourself when you are frustrated, like Tom.

In Rob's case, his old family dynamic taught him that an egalitarian, fluid sexual relationship with a woman would be too dangerous. The only way he could enjoy sex was to assure himself that the power issue was decided ahead of time. Unlike his childhood, when he didn't have the choice to submit, as a sexual adult, Rob would choose to be submissive, and he would consciously request the other person to be dominant.

Sexual addicts' patterns are similar to Tom's sexual habits. (See chapter 10.) In extreme cases, abusive families create criminals—sexual predators with a lack of empathy for others, who act out their rage by using sex to hurt others.

To experience sexual ecstasy with another person (in a relationship between peers) you must let go of the controls over your body, and allow an instinctive, biological process of arousal, continuing excitement, and orgasm to occur. You need to trust the other person to take good care of you, to listen to your wishes, and to give you sexual pleasure.

To be able to "let go" sexually, allowing yourself to feel unambivalently good about turning your body over to someone else to go into a sexual trance, you need to have a basic sense that you own yourself. You must feel secure that, in life, you are in control of *your* body and *your* wishes. Only then can it feel safe to make the *choice* to let go. Use the chapter exercises as well as the resources for this chapter (page 255) as a starting point for reclaiming your own power.

Exercises

Assess the Power Dynamics in Your Family

Take this quick test and reassess whether your family was primarily empathic, mixed empathic/controlling, or unempathic/controlling. If your family was primarily empathetic, you're less likely to have sexual problems involving control issues. However, if one or both of your parents were extremely domineering, or a mixture of domineering, neglectful, and occasionally empathic, it is likely that this has affected your sexuality in a negative way.

Test One

Answer the following questions.

	Yes	No
• I felt secure and unafraid in my family.	____	____
• I felt accepted by my parents.	____	____
• My parents met my basic needs.	____	____
• I felt my parents listened to my views and were willing to reconsider their decisions.	____	____
• I was allowed to control my own life in several areas that were important to me (for example, friends, food, beliefs, career).	____	____
• I was touched tenderly and appropriately by my parents.	____	____
• Physical violence was absent in my family.	____	____

If you answered yes to all of these questions, go on to the next chapter of the book. If not, go on to the following test.

Test Two

Answer the following questions.

	Yes	No
• I feel anxious whenever I have to see one or both of my parents.	____	____
• My family interactions left me feeling power-less and hopeless.	____	____
• Even as an adult, I worry if my parents disapprove of choices I am making in my own life.	____	____
• I find it hard to ask people for what I want.	____	____
• I have a hard time with people in authority.	____	____
• I find myself worried about who has more or less power in every relationship.	____	
• I believe that there is a one-up/one-down dynamic in most relationships.	____	____

	Yes	No
• I sometimes find myself in what feels like power struggles with people, even though I don't think I am really a competitive person.	____	____
• I just don't feel comfortable getting close to other people.	____	____
• I'm not sure that I really link sexuality and love.	____	____
• I have a lot of trouble letting go and being vulnerable in sexual relationships.	____	____

Now, looking at what you checked off, what bad lessons do you think you learned about power and relationships in your family? List them here.

_____

_____

_____

Having read this chapter and answered these questions, what are the ways in which you now think that your family power profile is interfering with your ability to connect closeness and sexuality?

_____

_____

_____

If you answered yes to more than three of the questions in the second test, issues of power and control are prominent in your relation ships and may cause problems in your sexual relationships. Continue with the following exercises.

My List of Fears About Control

Especially considering people with whom you are or want to be intimate, list your fears about how people currently in your life may try to control you:

_____

_____

_____

_____

_____

Reality-Test Your Power Fears

Looking at your responses thus far, list current fears about power dynamics that are based in past negative experiences with your family (for example, "If I give in to Jim on this then that'll be the beginning of a pattern where I never get my way."):

_____

_____

_____

_____

List your current fears about power dynamics that are based on your current life (may be based on fact: list the evidence for your belief next to your belief):

_____

_____

_____

_____

Reevaluate Your Fears

List three new ways you want to think about the power dynamics in the current relationships in your life:

1. _____

2. _____

3. _____

Do you have a pattern of avoiding contact? If so, list the times you have been afraid of getting close to another person and may have "missed the boat" on a relationship you wish you had pursued. If you need more space, use another piece of paper.

_____

_____

_____

_____

_____

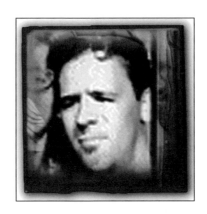

Chapter 7

Permission to Explore Self and Sexuality

Unless you give information and advice, your children are likely to remain sexually ignorant—and in danger.

—Martha and Howard Lewis, *Sex Education Begins at Home*

♦ Were you provided with an opportunity to learn about your sexuality within a nurturing and informing environment?

♦ Did your parents provide you with developmentally appropriate sexual information, without exposing you to information which made you feel overwhelmed or overstimulated?

♦ Did you feel comfortable asking your parents about sexuality, and did they answer you easily?

♦ Did the adults in your environment respect your privacy?

♦ Were you allowed to explore your own body in private?

♦ Did your parents give you the idea that your sexuality and your body were basically good?

♦ Did the adults in your environment model the appropriate expression of physical affection toward you, and yet not flaunt their own sexuality?

Most of us have been raised in families in which sexuality was not handled well, in one way or another. The theme of permission-giving within families is so important that it is discussed in almost every book about sexuality. Americans are particularly squeamish about the topic of sex.

Howard and Martha Lewis, authors of *Sex Education Begins at Home* (1983), make the point that discussions about sexuality are impossible in families where the general level of communication is low. If you couldn't talk to your parents about much of anything at all, you certainly couldn't talk to them about sex. In other families, communication might be high about other issues, but any discussion about sexuality or bodies is off-limits.

> Years ago, I was struck by a scene which occurred between a mother and her small daughter in the locker room of a large, public swimming pool in an upper-class suburb of Boston. The Disney movie *The Little Mermaid* had just come out, and the stores and the media were filled with images of the pretty mermaid, Ariel, who had two peach-colored scallop shells to cover her breasts, and a green fish tail.
>
> After the free swim period, the locker room was full of many, many women of all ages, sizes and descriptions, all walking around in various states of semi-nudity while getting themselves and their children dressed.
>
> A little girl began walking around in her underpants, with her hands cupped in the shape of seashells, one over each tiny nipple. "Look, Mommie, here are my boobies!" she said happily. The mother walked up to her, yanked her quite roughly by the arm, and harshly hissed, "Shut up. You don't say things like that."
>
> This little girl may or may not remember this actual incident, but it is certain that she absorbed the antisex, antibody message contained in this parent-child interaction. The likelihood of this little girl coming to her mom with later questions about sexuality is slim. It is not known for certain whether this mother was a good parent in other areas, or whether her parenting skills were poor in general.

Even giving and communicative parents can be poor communicators about sexuality. If your childhood and adolescent exploration of your sexual self was severely blocked and sanctioned (for example, you weren't allowed to talk about sex, think about sex, or touch your own body) and if you did not find a way to create your own freedom—to break out of your family's antisex prison through reading, peer experiences, or talking to another adult—you could not possibly have developed into an adult who feels that your sexuality is normal, pleasurable, and good.

> *I grew up in an atmosphere where there was no privacy. My privacy was never respected. I shared a bedroom with my grandmother until I was five or six. I was caught masturbating by her. She was disapproving, but I continued to masturbate and just was sneakier about it. My parents did not make a big deal about masturbating. Their message was: if you're going to do it, don't discuss it.*
>
> —Joan, 45

> *From ages four to six, I remember getting yelled and screamed at for getting caught masturbating, and I was punished regularly for any activity perceived as sexual.*
>
> —Howard, 32

> *My family openly discussed sex and sexuality during my adolescence. My mom always answered my questions accurately and to my satisfaction. As a result, I had lifelong comfort with sex and sexuality.*
>
> —Beth, 32

Sexual Curiosity

Being curious about sexuality as an infant, child, and adolescent is natural. Children have been seen touching their genitals, in utero, in ultrasound photographs. Infants only a few months old discover the pleasure of touching their genitals. In many families, children are considered asexual creatures, but parents' wishing doesn't make it so. Even if you don't remember instances of being sexually curious, consider these typical childhood vignettes:

- Two six-year-olds, a boy and a girl, are found playing doctor.

- A family gets a CD-ROM encyclopedia. The ten-year-old daughter and her same-aged friend run off, giggling enthusiastically, to use the computer. The mother walks in and finds them looking up "penis."

- A nine-year-old asks her mother if she and her husband "do it" and also if they do "cunnylingus" and fellatio.

- An eleven-year-old, watching TV with her brother, is asked to go to sleep so that the parents can have some time together. She responds, "We know you want to have sex. We want to stay up and watch TV in here. Why don't you just go in your room and have sex and let us stay out here and watch TV?"

- A twelve-year-old and her friend go to the state fair. There they see a giant horse. Mostly, they are fascinated by his giant penis.

At times, the media and the popular press make it seem as if the only problematic sexual climate is one in which there was overt sexual contact between parents and children. In actuality, families which ignore sexuality, as well as families which create a lot of sexual fear and shame can be almost as destructive—and are much more common in North America (Goldman and Goldman 1982).

Family Attitudes: Bolton, Morris, and MacEachron's Typology

One excellent typology of family attitudes toward sexuality comes from Bolton, Morris, and MacEachron's *Males At Risk* (1989). As you read about each of their categories, think about critical incidents from your own childhood and which model best represents your family of origin's sexual atmosphere.

"Ideal Environment"

In an ideal environment, parents understand that a child should be provided an opportunity to learn about their developing sexuality within a nurturing, supportive, and informative environment. They provide their child with appropriate, accurate, and useful sexual information at each new developmental stage. The significant adults in the child's environment model appropriate expression of sexuality and feelings.

"Predominantly Nurturing Environment"

In a predominantly nurturing environment, most of the conditions in the ideal environment are met, but there are some areas in which the support, education, and modeling are less than ideal. For instance, their child may be given more accurate than inaccurate information, but the usefulness of the information is hampered by some of the attitudes the parents express informally.

"Evasive Environment/Environmental Vacuum"

In an evasive environment, parents act as if sex does not exist. Children of evasive parents are given little or no accurate and useful information about sexual matters, or interpersonal relationships. These parents are totally uncomfortable talking about sex, and ignore their child's curiosity and questions about sexuality.

Well-meaning but overly modest parents believe that they are doing their children a favor by "protecting" them from learning about sexuality. In truth, sex-avoidant families truncate their children's ability to feel comfortable with sexuality as adults. Sex therapists find their offices filled with people who have been socialized not to even *think* about sex, therefore are unable to explore enough to know what they like sexually.

> When I was three or four years old, I was visiting a friend's house and was playing in the sandbox. I filled a cup with sand and then turned it over. I said, "That looks like a penis." My friend's mother angrily said that she was going to tell my mother that I had said this. Her reaction filled me with fear that I had done something horribly wrong, and I cried and pleaded with her not to tell.
>
> —Donna, 32

What was wrong with this three-year-old's simple observation about shapes and proper use of anatomical labels? If your parents were comfortable talking about sexuality, they did more than set up an open climate for discussion—they provided you with an opportunity to develop a vocabulary of sexual terms and a comfort in using these terms.

Children whose parents forbade the use of proper sexual terms, in the name of modesty or saintliness, can grow up to be adults who have neither the words nor the ease to talk with their partner about sexual problems.

> Sally and her husband, Jack, were both raised in homes where sexuality wasn't allowed or discussed. Neither of them had had much experience before their union. After ten years of marriage,

their sexual relationship was getting worse and worse. Sally appeared to be disgusted, and avoided sex.

After some exploration in sex therapy it became clear that Jack's lack of sexual experience caused him to be somewhat immature in the way he handled his body when approaching her. Sally, for her part, had a specific complaint that she had wanted to make a decade before, but which she was too embarrassed to talk about: Whenever they kissed, or danced, or he wanted to begin to make a sexual approach to her, Jack got an erection, which he poked into her.

In therapy, Sally learned to give Jack this sexual feedback and I modeled how she could do so. As soon as Sally was able to ask Jack to please move his erect penis to the side when he was just being affectionate, or they were dancing, Jack did so. Their sexual relationship improved.

At age nine, I remember asking my mother what sex was. My mother's response was,'Where did you hear that word?' When I told her I heard it in school, she said, 'Oh, You're too young to know about that now.' I never asked her about sex again.

—Robin, 25

My mother found it hard to explain sexuality issues. When talking about it, she would often use science books. Then she told me I would figure it out on my own.

—Lee, 48

Cindy came into sex therapy with her husband, Brad. Brad was glad that Cindy finally wanted to address the sexual problems which had upset him throughout their marriage: Cindy seemed totally unable to experience any physical pleasure during kissing, hugging, or more genital activities. Brad described her as "frozen." Cindy described herself as feeling "broken," and couldn't understand why she wasn't having what she considered to be the normal experiences of love and lust that she saw in the movies and TV and read about. And she was puzzled, too, because she had come from a loving family, without any kind of sexual incest or inappropriateness. "Why can't I get excited about sex?" she wondered.

In sex therapy, Cindy realized that although her parents were emotionally loving, they were not physically demonstrative at all. She also immediately recognized that they were evasive about sexuality. This gave her answers to the puzzle, but still didn't magically change how her body reacted to touch.

Cindy needed to reprogram herself that touch was something she liked, not just something she would do for Brad. She faithfully did six months of exercises to increase her comfort and good associations to touch (see the Resources and References sections at the back of this book). After all her work, Cindy remarked, "Now, when I breathe and relax and use the vibrator, I get so aroused it makes my toes curl. Wow, I can't even believe this is my same body!"

Ken, a responsible, married man in his forties, has suffered from lifelong retarded ejaculation during intercourse. "I have only ejaculated inside a woman two, or maybe three times, in my whole life," he commented. Ken was able to ejaculate if he masturbated, but when he and his wife wanted to become pregnant, this became an issue.

Ken grew up in a Southern home, one of three kids, the middle child between two girls. His mother was "a real Southern type" who didn't believe in "airing her dirty laundry to others."

Sexuality in any form was not discussed by either parent. His parents were extremely modest, and he wound up hearing "it isn't proper" in reference to a whole range of topics and behaviors.

During adolescence, Ken was a self-described "nerd" who hung out with a whole crowd of nerds. He was more interested in books than in girls, although he did masturbate a few times.

He lost his virginity the second year of college, but he couldn't ejaculate inside his first girlfriend.

"I never did an impulsive thing in my whole life," he said. In fact, when Ken was going out with girls in college he would masturbate ahead of time, so that he wouldn't feel too much sexual pressure.

In the course of discussing his ejaculatory inhibition, I asked Ken if he could urinate with his wife in the bathroom. He gave me a funny look, said it "just wasn't proper," and then confessed to feelings of irritation if he was in the presence of a man who was casual about closing the bathroom door while urinating. As we discussed his life, Ken began to connect his physical inhibitions, learned in his family, with his sexual problem.

"Permissive Environment"

In a permissive environment, parents adopt a well-meaning, completely open and unexamined philosophy about a child's exposure to sexual matters. They may provide a child with accurate sexual information, but the information may be too much for a child's mind to process. Appropriate boundaries for sexual activities are missing. For instance, a child may be exposed to nudity or adult sexual behaviors which are too stimulating for them to see.

Overly permissive parents don't empathize with their children's changing needs for modesty or privacy. They don't understand that it is possible to overwhelm a child, through an openness—for instance, with sexual talk or nudity—that can feel embarrassing or repulsive.

Throughout my childhood, and even into my adolescence, my father walked around in the nude after his shower. I thought it was disgusting, really.

—Toni, 69

"Negative Environment"

In a negative environment parents burden their child with misinformation, negative attitudes, and fear—telling their child that sex is bad, evil, abnormal, harmful, a sign of moral weakness, or something to be avoided. Their child is given very little accurate information, and any attempts to gain information about sexuality on their own is blocked or punished.

Exploring one's body is totally forbidden, and children are emotionally or physically punished when they try to do it. They may learn to associate sexual feelings with shame and aversive consequences.

My mother really hated sex. And she was always complaining to us about it. When I was growing up, their bed was against my wall, and they'd have sex, and I could hear the bed slamming into the wall, and hear my mother's voice, weary, saying, "Oh John," like she wanted him to stop. It really was nauseating. It's such a bad memory.

And now, she still dumps her sexual issues on me. When I asked her how the cruise they took was, she commented, "Oh, Jessie, I couldn't have any fun. Your father kept bothering me, trying to get me to stay in the cabin and do it, every few hours." I wish she'd deal with her own problems. I have enough trouble feeling good about sexuality myself.

—Jessica, 40

John came into therapy with his wife, Jenny. Jenny complained that John was uncomfortable with touch, and that he was so inhibited sexually that their relationship was not fun for her.

John's religious parents had taught him that sexual expression was wrong, and that masturbation was a sin. His parents used fear to scare him away from experimentation.

"I was told that my soul was like a milk bottle. If I was good (i.e., not masturbating) I was white. But each sin made my soul a little blacker, as if the milk in the bottle turned black. That image scared me. Every time I wanted to experiment, I feared I would go to hell."

Needless to say, John was too frightened to masturbate or experiment sexually. John grew up to believe that only "dirty girls" really liked sex. He couldn't integrate the fact that his "good" wife, Jenny, had sexual desire, and he didn't feel comfortable acting lustful and erotic with her.

Martha came into sex therapy because of an inability to become aroused, even though she loved her husband and was attracted to him. In looking for the source of her inhibitions she remembered several incidents in which she was yelled at for anything considered sexual. In one instance, at age seven, she was caught rubbing her pelvis against a couch and was yelled at so severely that she has never tried masturbating since. In another instance, her mother slapped her hand when she reached for a sanitary napkin to investigate what it was.

Martha's mother was extremely squeamish about menstruation, as well as unenthusiastic about intercourse. She felt unclean when she was menstruating had hated using pads but told her girls that she didn't want to use tampons, because it was "putting something 'in there.'" Martha was taught to feel uncomfortable even having a vagina.

As an adult, Martha feels completely unsexy during her menstrual period and jumps back if her husband touches her when she is wearing a sanitary pad.

Dr. Leonore Tiefer (1979) has assessed that the leading source of adult female sexual difficulty lies in the scanty and negative information girls have been given about their genitals. Boys are taught that they have a penis and testicles—they learn that they must handle the penis to urinate; girls are often taught only that they *have* a vagina, which is the reproductive organ—they are rarely taught about the clitoris, which is the organ which feels sexual pleasure. In addition, they are not taught any circumstances in which it is acceptable to touch their genitals.

For boys and girls between eight and fourteen, sex education is extremely important. Traditionally, preparation for puberty in American society has been gravely inadequate: it is a common experience for boys to think that their first nocturnal emission means they have a horrible disease; girls who are not taught about menstruation often believe the same thing. Parents who are not comfortable answering questions about sexual development and sexuality don't stick around to see what questions remain. When you were this age, what information did you want and need? Did you get it? Or did you learn misinformation from your parents?

> Geri remembers her mother explaining to her about menstruation. However, through the explication she was given, she concluded that this bloody process was something which would happen to a girl once in her life.

Your parents' attitude toward nudity or your genitals, their discomfort with discussing sexuality, or their belief that sex is dirty can hinder you by creating negative adult attitudes toward masturbation, oral sex, intercourse during menstruation, and varied foreplay.

As in childhood, the young person asks questions and picks up the emotional climate of the answer, thus is less likely to ask questions that the instructor clearly does not feel comfortable answering. During preadolescence, the parents' reactions to the youngster's budding sexual interests predict what the interactions will be later on, when the hints become demands.

Adults might make fun of children's sexuality and act like it's foolish and premature. They also may show their anxiety by being suspicious of sexual activities. Other parents may react positively to the "signs of budding pubescence" (Tiefer 1979, 53). Their reactions depend to a large extent on the cultural environment as well as the parent's own relation to *their* sexuality.

"Seductive Environment"

Children of seductive sexual environments are given messages that one of their parents is interested in them in sexual ways, though overt sexual contact does not occur. Information about sexuality may be presented in ways that are arousing to the child sexually, rather than in ways that are informative. The mixed physical and verbal messages and the unstable nature of the sexual feelings in such an environment disrupt the natural unfolding of that child's own sexual development.

> The seductive environment in which Johann grew up contributed to his erectile dysfunction with women. Johann's mother, Dorothy, drank so much that by the time he was twelve, his father had left the house, leaving Johann and his younger sister to fend for themselves. Dorothy herself had come from a disordered family background, and she had neither the emotional nor the intellectual capacity to think about what her children needed in terms of structure.
>
> After the divorce, she just fell apart. She leaned on Johann emotionally, and tried several times to get him to lie down on her bed and hold and comfort her while she cried. Johann had very mixed feelings about this behavior, and he did it a few times. As he got older, Dorothy would dress so provocatively around him that he would have to go into his bedroom and masturbate to get rid of the sexual tension. He really hated her for this, but he also felt guilty that he felt such repugnance toward his own mother. He knew that emotionally, she was weak. He didn't believe she meant him any harm.
>
> When Johann became an adult, he struggled with the kind of woman he would choose for a partner. He eventually married a woman he thought was more competent than his mother. She didn't drink and was a good wife and mother. However, he had off-again, on-again troubles with lack of desire, which frustrated his wife. As she got more assertive in asking for sex, Johann's problem turned into one of erectile difficulty.
>
> In sex therapy, he discovered that his associations to sex, and to his wife wanting sex, were old connections of shame and disgust at Dorothy's general inadequacy as a person, her out-of-control sexuality, her seduction toward him, and his shame and guilt at masturbating using his mother's image as a sex object.

Norma felt disgusted by sex with her husband, whom she loved, and she couldn't figure it out. Her parents loved her, and they were affectionate. She knew that she hadn't been sexually abused. Norma's life looked perfect. She had gone to the best schools, had lessons in every conceivable sport and art form, and had been given a sports car as soon as she got her driver's license. What had happened in Norma's seemingly charmed life to make her feel "icky" about sex? She had also been raised in a seductive environment by her father, Brad. Brad was unusually handsome and charming, and all of her friends had a crush on him. But as she got older, her dad's over-interest in her physical development and his oversexualized affection left her feeling uneasy.

"When I think of it now, it was kind of sick. He called me his little 'puss,' which all my brothers teased me about. He was way too interested in what my bra size was, and a little too caught up in how pretty I looked in my bathing suit. There were times he kissed me on the lips, which really grossed me out. And there were times when I felt like I was supposed to replace my mother, like when he took me as his 'date' to the ballet, because my mother didn't really like ballet."

The feelings of inappropriateness that Norma had felt about her father's sexual attraction to her had been unknowingly transferred to her husband.

"Overtly Sexual Environment"

In such an environment, there *is* overtly sexualized contact between a parent and child, or the parent may encourage inappropriate sexual contact among the children. The sexual information that is provided to the child is for the purpose of furthering sexual contact or sexual exploitation.

And so from about ages five to ten, I wound up going over to my grandfather's every week, so he could molest me. I just shut it out, and I went on with the rest of my life. Thank God he died when I was ten, so that the abuse stopped. But even after I've talked about it, and it makes me feel better to understand it, I still can't figure out why I acted so passively later in my teenage years, when that neighbor came over periodically and did all that sexual stuff to me.

—Shirley, 24

The most dramatic damage to children's developing sexuality is done by families in which any overt sexual contact—which constitutes abuse—occurs. Common issues revolve around safety, empowerment, stigmatized sexuality, inappropriate shame and guilt, negative associations to sexuality, as well as trust, assertiveness, and communication skills. If you have been a victim of sexual abuse, it is important to address your trauma directly (see the Resources section for recommended books on the subject of surviving sexual abuse).

Give Yourself Permission

Growing up in a warm, loving family which avoids discussing sex, in and of itself, isn't a major stumbling block to adult sexuality. Considering that many adult North Americans have grown up in sex-avoidant families, this is a lucky break for most of us. If you have had excellent parenting in all of the other spheres, it is likely that you are assertive enough and social enough to gain your sexual socialization and knowledge outside your family, though books, discussions, or courses.

In loving families, it is when sex avoidance and sexual negativity from parents combine with stumbling blocks in other important developmental stages that major problems occur. For instance, if families don't touch, or don't do a good job of flirting and making the child feel like an attractive boy or girl *and*, in addition, don't recognize or discuss human sexuality, children won't grow up to picture themselves as the object of anyone else's sexual desire. In less loving families, the combination of negative sexual family environments combined with other deficient rearing with regard to self-esteem, body image, and/or power can create more severe sexual problems, which may be even more difficult to overcome.

If your family's attitude about sexuality was negative or evasive, you must now give yourself permission to get the information you need, and to explore your sexual self. If there was a sexually seductive or overly sexual atmosphere, excellent resources to overcome your feelings of shame, guilt, and disgust are available. See the Resources list for this chapter at the end of the book.

Exercises

Now, looking again at Bolton, Morris, and MacEachron's typology, list some critical memories you have of your sexual upbringing and which category you believe characterizes your family of origin's sexual environment.

_____

_____

_____

List three negative beliefs about sexuality which you absorbed in your family.

_____

_____

_____

Now write three correcting beliefs.

1. _____

2. _____

3. _____

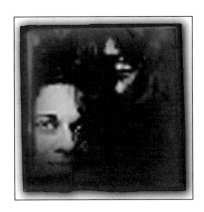

Chapter 8

Becoming a Social Person

If you realize the advantage of exposing children at an early age to play with other children, you also recognize the importance of teaching your child to share, to play cooperatively, and to inhibit aggressive behavior . . . . Rather than leave such important matters to chance, you can teach your child some specific behaviors which will make positive social experiences possible for many years.

—Doris Durrell, *Starting Out Right: Essential Parenting Skills for Your Child's First Seven Years*

♦ **Do you feel competent socially?**

♦ **Do (or did) your parents have friends?**

♦ **Did your parents help you to establish and maintain friendships as a child?**

♦ **Were you liked by your peers as a child?**

♦ **Are you well liked now?**

♦ **Do you have a few friends, people you trust with personal information about you?**

♦ **Can you ask people for what you need?**

♦ **Do you know how to have fun and to play?**

How well did your parents socialize you? Did they train you so that you developed the qualities that make you able to live comfortably with others? Did they teach you the skills you need to live with others and to take part in the social life around you? Did they help you learn how to make and keep friends?

One of the areas people don't think about when considering their difficulties in sexual adjustment is their past experience—good or bad—with peer friendship. While biological maturity is physically based, sexuality unfolds within a social context.

Healthy sexuality is based in trust, communication, and relationship. How can you be intimate and trust someone else with your *body* if you don't even know whether they can understand your thoughts and feelings? Your childhood friendships taught you to connect to, communicate with, and trust a person outside your immediate family.

Social Skills

In your early years and middle childhood, your parents were the major influence on your social skills development—and there are many reasons why your parents may have failed in this task. For example, parents who are openly rejecting, neglectful, or abusive create children who are socially isolated and afraid to trust anyone.

> *Now I understand myself better, why I act and feel the way I do. I understand that the issue isn't just intercourse, it's being guarded, getting hurt, feeling threatened, and it's about trust.*
> —Charles, 42

> *I found I couldn't believe that this new friend, Adena, actually liked me. It really struck me how bad my mother screwed me up in this area of my life. It's sad that my mother could debilitate me like this by rejecting me like she did. I feel such powerlessness with other people sometimes. The sense of self-worth and strength I have alone just does not translate when I am dealing with other people and depending on them personally. . . . I figure when they find out about the struggling part of me that they don't see right away they will, of course, get frustrated with that and not understand it and leave me.*
> —Elizabeth, 30

Some of you may have had good parents who had financial or medical problems, and felt overwhelmed as if they could barely keep their heads above water. Parents such as these did the best they could, they just couldn't cope with helping their children with friendships.

Some other, basically decent, parents may have been too disorganized to help you develop and maintain friendships, lacking the energy to keep track of your friends and go the extra mile to make dates for you to play with friends, set up birthday parties, have sleepovers, or feed and care for extra visitors to the house. Or, you may have grown up in a home where a parent's relationship with you met that parent's need for a sympathetic ear or companionship. Your parent might not have wanted to share you with others.

Some of you had attentive and loving parents in other ways, but for some reason they had difficulty helping you to be social. For instance, your parents may be shy or have poor social skills themselves. Or a parent may be unaware of the importance of encouraging you to relate to others outside the family, only valuing your intellectual growth, or some other aspect of your development.

To focus on how your childhood friendships—or lack thereof—connects to your adult sexuality, think for a moment about the significance to a child of having a best friend. Children totally depend on their parents when they are tiny. But when their emotional needs for trust and caring and empathy have been met adequately in the family, children begin to trust other people and look to them for fun, support, and companionship. Some children, magically, at the age of six, seven, eight, nine, or ten, find a soul mate outside of the family—a best friend.

Did you have a best friend when you were a child? If you did, then you remember wanting to spend all of your time with this new person, playing, talking, sharing feelings, exploring. The success of this new relationship taught you that love and support was to be had outside the family, as well as within it. If you do not remember having a best friend, your parents may have failed to assist in your social development—and you may find yourself petrified to rely on others.

> *It must be nice to be able to ask other people for what you need. My mother always told me to fight my own battles and that she couldn't help me. The times I went to her crying or asked for her help, which were often, she always let me down and it hurt really badly. It's devastating when I think about it.*
>
> —Elizabeth, 30

Creating socially successful and unafraid kids takes much more focus and energy than just creating a trusting baby and child. Your parents needed to be socially unafraid and competent themselves—high-functioning, energetic, sophisticated, consistent, and empathic—to teach you the complicated ways of thinking and acting to insure you success with your peers, in early childhood and beyond.

Parents also have to be emotionally generous, relatively well organized, and not depressed in order to create a family milieu conducive to older children's friendships. Creating socially competent children is a prolonged, major task, even for healthy parents in a long-term, stable relationship.

From the Beginning

You can't develop the skills to successfully relate to another human being sexually without a firm foundation of general social skills. Beginning as young as age one and one-half, your parents should have begun to teach you how to be aware of the other people around you, and how to interact with others in a pleasant, constructive way.

Dr. Doris Durrell (1989), a child psychologist, has written a brilliant, extremely detailed, how-to book for parents of young children. Dr. Durrell's prescription for good parenting explains why some of us may lack social skills. She insists that parents of young children, beginning at least by the child's second year, must actively teach cooperative play and inhibition of aggression. According to Dr. Durrell, your parents *should* have provided minute-to-minute, close supervision of all social interactions with other children. They should have modeled the way you should have acted, using both words and motions. Dr. Durrell believes that children younger than three years should never be left to their own devices to "figure out" sharing and collaboration.

Did this happen in your family? Many of us grew up in families where parents were tired or depressed, life was chaotic, and there just were too many children to parent each child this diligently.

Age Three to Six

According to Dr. Durrell, by the age of three, children are much more interested in being with other children and actually are able to interact with them, not just play in a parallel fashion. By three and a half, children are capable of a real emotional attachment to another child.

If your parents supervised you and modeled good social skills in their own interactions with others, certain sociable abilities that you need as an adult developed when you were between the ages of three and six, including finding out how to exchange information with others, discovering how to establish common ground, learning to disclose feelings, and mastering conflict resolution (i.e., learning to share and how not to be aggressive).

Were you well liked as a child? By four years of age, some children are well liked and others are significantly less successful with other kids. Durrell points out that a child who is rejected socially (for instance, the ones who can't share equipment, disrupt classroom activities, can't work and play cooperatively, are angry, or are physically or verbally abusive to others) will probably continue to be rejected for several years.

If you didn't learn social skills early, you may have been rejected by others, leading to social—and then sexual—insecurity as adults. Boys who are rejected as children sometimes become increasingly aggressive over time, creating a cycle of continuing aggression and rejection.

Tim was lonely, had poor self-esteem, and had never had a sexual connection to another person until he "fell in love" with a first cousin who was pregnant out of wedlock. His strange relationship with his cousin was causing much consternation in his family.

At twenty-three, Tim was of below normal intelligence, and in some ways, he didn't even have the social skills of a four-year-old. He felt that people didn't like him and picked on him.

Tim's mother was uneducated and drank a lot during his childhood. She expressed puzzlement about his social failure. At the same time, she told the therapist that up until kindergarten, Tim had no experience playing with children other than his sister. Tim's mother explained that Tim had had a lot of ear infections as a small child, and she couldn't take the risk of him "catching anything" from other children. So she literally kept him in their yard for the first few years of his life, while she stayed in the house, doing her chores.

When Tim finally entered kindergarten, he immediately got into trouble. He didn't know how to share and he behaved aggressively. The teachers told her about Tim's social problems, but Tim's mother didn't know what to do about them, so she did nothing.

Tim became the scapegoated, rejected child, a role he had throughout his childhood and adolescence. He was able to "fall in love" with his cousin because, having known her all his life, she was not emotionally threatening.

Unfortunately Tim's parents did not catch the obvious signals that he needed some extra help in relating to his peers. In therapy, Tim was able to address his deficit. In addition, Tim realized that socially desirable skills which may not have been learned in childhood can be learned at any age.

Age Seven to Nine

By eight or nine years old, many children like to spend time together, go on trips together, play games, sleep over, explore the surrounding neighborhood, and hang out. Children with this kind of friendship network have truly learned the pleasures of being with peers, and the give and take of relationships. For parents of these well-connected kids, this means that not only are their own children tromping around the house, asking for things, making noise and messes and eating food, but so is a revolving cast of other kids. If you didn't have many friends at that age, because of the way your family functioned, you might feel a little awkward or shy socially now.

Boundaries

If your parents came from homes in which the family boundaries were fluid, where they themselves enjoyed the chaos of having lots of friends around, then chances are, you were allowed the same freedom. But if your parents came from rigidly structured homes, where no one else ever ate or slept over, they may have felt invaded by your friends, and they may not have encouraged you to reach out to others.

Even if your house wasn't like this, you might have been lucky enough to be friends with someone whose parents treated you like family, and let you use their own house as a "home away from home."

My own parents were so uptight that I never could have kids over. I don't know how I could have survived without Donny's parents. He was in my neighborhood and was my best friend throughout my childhood. From about the time I was nine on, I lived over there. I could go in their refrigerator, sleep over any time I wanted on the weekend. I could talk to his dad and his mom. About anything. I even went on vacation with them once. They were the first people outside my family I ever learned to trust. Donny's house was where I learned that the outside world is a safe and friendly place. I really felt close to the whole family. Even now, as an adult, when I go back to my hometown, I always visit Donny's parents.

—Tom, 35

Intervening

At certain times, parental empathy, careful listening, good judgment and belief in the value of friendship are critical in helping children succeed with their peers. This is particularly true when a child is hurt by something minor a very good friend said or did.

Left to their own devices, children will handle this situation in unproductive ways—with open aggression, or by rejecting a child who temporarily hurt their feelings. As a result of a recent spat, for example, a child may want not to invite a good friend to an upcoming birthday party. A wise parent will empathize with the child about having her feelings hurt, but insist that the child invite her good friend to the party nonetheless, based on the history of the relationship. By the time the party occurs, the two will probably be harmonious again, and a lesson has been learned in the value of friendship, value, and trust. Do you remember if your parent had the skills or energy to intervene like this in your childhood relationships?

Some parents make the mistake of undermining their child's trust in others by teaching their child to be suspicious of other people. Still others overtly discourage friendship, telling their children that others who make overtures to them are not to be trusted, and that people outside the family will invariably let them down. Distrustful messages pull children away from relationships with others by creating fear of betrayal, or making the child question why anyone outside the family might want to be friends. For example:

See, I knew Rachel couldn't be trusted. Don't invite her to your birthday party, and just stop being friends with her.

Blood is thicker than water, you know.

What do you think she wants you to go there and play for?

You might think he is your friend, but when the chips are down, Karl, you can really only trust your family. We're the only ones who will stand by you when the going gets tough.

Still other parents don't have any intimates themselves. They do not model the advantages of having their own confidantes.

I have to say that I can't remember my mother having a single good friend. She always told me it was best to keep to yourself, that other people gossiped, and not to let anyone know my business. Even now, as an adult, if I talk to her about my friends (and I have had a hard time learning to trust enough to even have friends), she makes suspicious comments that let me know she thinks relationships are a bad thing.

—Carrie, 37

Neglect

Severely neglectful, unempathic families—where children's basic needs for trust, empathy, and warmth are not met—inevitably fall short in teaching children socialization skills. If you grew up in a neglectful family, a whole chain of events, starting in early childhood, conspired to make it difficult for you to trust others.

Your self-esteem was impacted, because you didn't feel cared for. No one listened to you. You may have stopped trying to ask for what you wanted because the situation seemed so hopeless, so your communication skills suffered.

When secure adults communicate, they keep talking back and forth until each one understands what the other is trying to say. This builds the basis of trust and understanding necessary to form a safe nonsexual relationship, which is a condition for moving on to a healthy sexual relationship. Children from neglectful homes never learn this back-and-forth communication process because parents don't take the time to listen. They give up on expecting that others will care about them, listen, and take the time to really understand.

Thankfully, as an adult, you can take the risk of trying to get others to really understand you. And it will pay off in feeling much more socially competent, and much more valued, by other people.

I have been telling my husband and my best friend a lot more about what's going on inside of me lately, and that has felt good. It makes me feel closer to both of them, and they are telling me that they like to feel needed. Plus they'll think of things in their lives that are similar or whatever, and so we talk about that as well. I have been really trying, when I get to a point where one of them might say something, and I can tell that they didn't get what I meant, to go one step further, and to pursue it and clarify what I meant, rather than dropping it, which is what I find I tend to do. It really works. It feels wonderful to have them be able to understand me better.

—Janet, 45

If your parents were neglectful, they probably didn't have the sophistication, time, or energy to take you to preplanned play times with others when you were a little child. You may have felt sorry for one of your parents and stuck around the house to look after them.

By fourth grade or so, when other children typically begin to strike out on their own and have close friendships, independently engineered playtimes together, and sleepovers, you may have opted out, because you didn't want others to meet your parents or see what was actually going on in your disordered house.

I feel like I got through my childhood in some kind of numb state. I can't remember much of anything. Dad was drinking all of the time, and some of the time he was really out of control, yelling at us kids and at Mom. I don't remember any affection from either parent.

I know that Mom was doing the best that she could, but she didn't seem to be able to handle anything. She never should have had four kids. None of us could count on her for anything. She didn't even remember our birthdays half the time! It was pointless to ask for anything you wanted; you wouldn't get it anyway. She'd forget you even asked. She didn't believe that children had real problems. She only believed that her problems were real. To this day, I don't really trust that anyone would take my needs or problems seriously. I find it difficult to get close to people.

School was hell. No one cared about how I did academically, so I didn't try hard. I felt terrible about myself. I was skinny, I hated my curly hair, and I had these terrible, buck teeth. I was teased a lot in junior high, but of course, Mom didn't take my upset seriously. Braces were out of the question.

We never went anywhere as a family. We never had the money, and she couldn't plan anything. None of us were encouraged to have any friends. We were supposed to play with each other, but my older brothers mostly just tortured me with their teasing. I really withdrew all the way through junior high and high school.

There was no discussion of sexuality or of relationships, period.

Later on, I got a job as a secretary and moved out. It was hard to feel confident in the outside world. Some of the other girls in the office seemed interested in being friends, but I was frightened of rejection and stayed aloof. I had this really strong feeling that there were some "rules" of knowing how to start and maintain friendships, and that everyone knew them except me.

I let my hair grow out, and men started paying attention to me, but I was petrified. I finally began to date a very kind man who worked in the office. We got very serious, and he wants to marry me. We have been dating for two years. He has been so kind to me that I basically trust him, but on some level I am holding back. I have put off all my longing and needs for so long that I guess I'm scared of being hurt if I let myself open up. Sex is a big problem. I can't relax and enjoy touching, and although we have intercourse, I can't seem to get excited enough to have an orgasm.

—Claudia, 36

Parents Who Are Overly Possessive

Some parents, for one reason or another, subtly or actively prevent their children from connecting to others outside the family, in order to inappropriately strengthen the parent-child bond.

Geoff came into sexual therapy because he was afraid of women and couldn't perform sexually. Geoff grew up in a household with a loving, but isolated and alcoholic mother. His father was verbally abusive to his mother and not available emotionally. Geoff was terrified for his mother and felt that he wanted to protect her.

Geoff's mother was miserable in her marriage, but she was afraid to leave it. Geoff was the light of her life. She loved to talk to him about art, literature, and history, even when he was small.

Geoff's mother was quite withdrawn. She lived in her house with the blinds drawn and wouldn't let Geoff invite any children over to play. She wanted him to come directly home from school, as well, and not to go to anyone else's house to visit. She wanted him for herself. As a ten-year-old, he once broke Mother's rules and went off exploring a quarry with some buddies. Mother called the police and punished him severely. He felt guilty.

Over time, Geoff's social skills suffered. He could only play with a few neighborhood kids, and as the years went by, he was playing with younger and younger children. He no longer felt competent to play with his peers.

By the time he went off to college, he had had absolutely no experience dating. Women were attracted to him, but Geoff was so unskilled and unpracticed at making conversations and getting close to other people that he was terrified of being with them. When he finally tried to have intercourse with a woman he liked a lot, his anxiety was so high that he could not perform sexually, a problem that persisted for many years. Geoff's lack of friendship skills directly impacted on his ability to express himself sexually.

Parents Who Move a Lot

Some families make it very difficult for the developing child to form and keep friendships, because they move from one area of the country to the other frequently. This puts the child in the unenviable position of being the new kid on the block, feeling left out or picked on, over and over again.

> . . . *so we moved all the time, and then my mother moved us twice after they got divorced. That's too bad, really, since maybe if we had lived in one place awhile, I might have found other adults—family, or friends' families or something—to talk to. It really contributed to all of us ending up being such isolated people.*
>
> —Betty, 55

Family Secrets

Some families have secrets, like spousal or child-battering, or alcohol or drug abuse. There are many negative aspects of growing up in homes like these, including bad associations to trust, lack of empathy, or lowered self-esteem. The social implications are substantial.

If your family had these kinds of secrets, you may have missed out on a whole range of important experiences with peers. Your communication skills suffered because you didn't dare share what your day-to-day life was like, because you were ashamed. You couldn't bring friends home because you were afraid of what your friends would see. You couldn't attend parties because your parents weren't willing or able to get you the appropriate clothes or buy needed gifts.

> *I stopped bringing friends home in about the sixth grade, after this one episode where my dad came home drunk on a Friday afternoon and started screaming at me and throwing things around. No one in school knew that my father drank. My family looked normal. It was our little secret. After that time, I was so scared that my friend would tell everyone at school what she had seen; I worried about it all weekend long. I never had anyone over again.*
>
> —Tammy, 28

Parents Who Don't Value Friendships

Some parents are naïve about the value of friendship, putting greater valuation on other aspects of your development, such as on intellectual achievement, or the nurturing of a great musical or sports ability. If your parents were like this, but you were innately skilled socially, you may grow up to feel quite comfortable having friends anyway. However, if you were naturally shy or very tied to pleasing your parents, you may be very skilled in whatever the valued trait in your family was, but be insecure socially and sexually.

Parents Who Are Workaholics

Families, by example, either teach that it is okay to play or that it is not okay to play. You need to feel good about playing in order to enjoy sex as an adult.

Some very nice families overtly or covertly teach their offspring that it is not all right to play until *everything* else conceivable which might be accomplished has been done. Kids from families like this aren't allowed to "goof off with friends" very often, because there is too much work to be done.

They don't have good memories of hanging out with their friends as kids—the easy give and take of joking around, with nothing to do and no place to go. As adults, they feel guilty if they set aside time to have fun. Self-esteem equals continuous hard work.

Such kids were socialized to be super-responsible. Often, they grew up in families which valued physical work but didn't value physical touch. As children, work was seen as the measure of their self-worth. Their parents worked hard, too, viewing the drudgery as the measure of what good and reliable parents they were. There wasn't much unstructured, relaxed time as a family—no drives without destinations, no lazy days playing at the beach.

> *My father could never stand to go on vacations. Any time we'd go on holiday as a family, he'd always find an excuse to leave. He'd say, "Damn, it's raining. I'm not just going to hang around here, wasting time. We're packing up and going home!" And so we curtailed every vacation.*
>
> —Curtis, 49

When children who were taught all about the value of work but nothing about the value of play grow into adulthood, they don't feel comfortable taking time out of their busy lives to be sexual. After all, there is nothing productive about sex, unless your job that month is to make a baby.

They literally can't rest until every last chore in their home and yard is done. If they don't accomplish what there is to be done, they don't feel like good people. But at the end of the day, this leaves them too spent emotionally and too tired physically to connect to their loved one.

For two adults who care about each other, having fun together is a way to connect emotionally, to be close, to loosen the boundaries between you. Super-responsible but humorless people are good citizens, and good working fellows, but not good sexual partners.

If you were raised in a workaholic home, relaxation may equal anxiety! Perhaps you feel awkward with free time. ("I don't know what we'd do if we didn't work on a project together. I guess maybe we could go to a movie.") Maybe free time together with a partner is "boring." If so, the boredom probably stems from a lack of warm childhood memories of unwinding with mother, father, siblings, or friends.

When you have free time, do you clean the gutters, change the oil in the car, clean the oven, or vacuum the closets? If you recognize yourself in this description, force yourself to reexamine your views on work and play, and begin to put playful, relaxing encounters higher on your priority list.

In fact, for many of us, life is so hectic that the only way to find time to connect sexually is literally to schedule in sex/play time. So the question is, do you feel too guilty to schedule in some fun?

Improving Your Social Skills

We've reviewed many ways in which families can help or hurt our adult social and sexual competency. What is terribly sad is that the sense of social awkwardness which can be formed in childhood lingers on, into adulthood, making forays into friendship and into sexual relationships seem too scary to consider. Look at the following list of children's socially desirable skills from Dr. Doris Durell's book, *Starting Out Right* (1989, 238):

Children's Socially Desirable Behavior

- asks questions

- gives information

- invites child to visit

- makes suggestions for play

- gives praise to friends

- expresses appreciation

- plays cooperatively

- shares

- takes turns

- compromises

- is agreeable to friends' ideas, rather than argumentative or bossy

- offers alternative ideas when disagreeing

- successfully enters ongoing play

- can initiate play

- communicates well—waits for and responds to friends' comments.

Reprinted with permission.

You will see that they are not very different from the skills an adult needs to succeed with others socially and sexually.

These abilities are mastered by practice. A child who feels that she has become socially skillful integrates that image of herself as a success with people into her developing sense of self-esteem. A child who hasn't had enough chance to practice and become competent with friends develops a sense of being a social dud, which translates into sexuality as well.

If you feel like a social dud, you can improve your own social skills now. You can learn to trust, and to develop and deepen your communication and your friendship with others. These proficiencies can be learned in adulthood. And it's worth trying, even though it takes a great deal of courage.

Exercises

Assess Your Family of Origin's Social Environment

Read the following statements and decide if they pertain to your family of origin, circling "Y" for "yes," "S" for "sometimes," or "N" for "no":

1. My mother could be depended on to meet most of my needs. Y S N

2. My father could be depended on to meet most of my needs. Y S N

3. When I made myself vulnerable and asked for what I needed in my family, I was listened to and responded to. Y S N

4. My mother made me think and feel that others, outside the family, would like me and value my friendship. Y S N

5. My father made me think and feel that others, outside the family, would like me and value my friendship. Y S N

6. I knew that my mother was glad that I had friends outside the family. Y S N

7. I knew that my father was glad that I had friends outside the family. Y S N

8. I felt okay about bringing friends into my home. Y S N

9. I was allowed to go to my friends' houses to play. Y S N

10. When I was younger, my parents went out of their way to help me have friends (made birthday parties, made play dates). Y S N

11. My parents were interested in my friendships and helped me figure things out when I was upset or disappointed by a friend. Y S N

12. My mother accepted my friends. Y S N

13. My father accepted my friends. Y S N

14. My parents actively taught me that trusting and depending on friends was a good thing to do. Y S N

15. My parents taught me that when a friend hurt me, I should try to work it out and forgive them. Y S N

16. My mother had friends (outside the family) she connected to and depended upon. Y S N

17. My father had friends (outside the family) he connected to and depended upon. Y S N

18. My parents believed that having fun was worthwhile. Y S N

19. My parents believed that having fun *with other people* was worthwhile. Y S N

20. Neither of my parents was jealous about my friendships, nor overly possessive of me. Y S N

If you had mostly Ss, friendship-based problems are most likely not a problem for you in your sexual development. If you had many Ss and Ns, complete the following exercises.

Sexuality/Socialization: An Inventory

Looking at your responses to the list in the first exercise, you can now identify several problematic aspects of what you were taught about friendship. List here the three beliefs or behavior patterns you learned in your family which you need to address.

1. Belief _____

   How it affected my sexual expression _____

   _____

2. Belief _____

   How it affected my sexual expression _____

   _____

3. Belief _____

   How it affected my sexual expression _____

   _____

Challenge Your Beliefs

List here what you now believe to be the three most important, healthy beliefs about friendships which will counteract the problematic beliefs about friendships you've previously held. Make sure the new messages are stated as positives. (If you are having trouble constructing them, look back at the first exercise.)

1. Healthy Belief _____

   _____

   How will your social and sexual interactions change if you believe this?

   _____

   _____

2. Healthy Belief _____

   _____

   How will your social and sexual interactions change if you believe this?

   _____

   _____

3. Healthy Belief _____

   _____

   How will your social and sexual interactions change if you believe this?

   _____

   _____

Thought-Stopping

Make a little card up for yourself listing your three most destructive thoughts or beliefs about friendship, along with the three counteracting thoughts. Keep it with you throughout the day. When you find yourself repeating the negative beliefs to yourself, consciously stop yourself and replace the negative thought or belief about friendship with a positive, encouraging thought or belief.

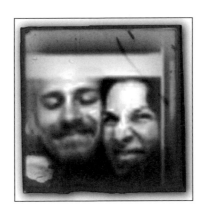

Chapter 9

Masturbation and Fantasy

Masturbation is one of the most common sexual expressions during the childhood years.

—Robert Crooks and Karla Baur, *Our Sexuality*

♦ **Did you fantasize or masturbate as you were growing up?**

♦ **How did you feel about it? Did you feel guilty, fine, or ambivalent?**

♦ **Did you use masturbation, compulsively, to soothe yourself because your life at home was frustrating and upsetting?**

Masturbation and fantasy play an important role in sexual development. In the very first few years of life, many girls and boys discover the pleasures of genital stimulation, if parents permit this. Later in childhood, masturbation provides a way of getting to know one's body, an experience of linking genital touch with pleasure, and a concrete sense of owning one's body and its functions. In adolescence, masturbation provides a way to acquaint and reacquaint oneself with one's constantly changing body and a substantive self-knowledge of what feels good sexually. Once the body has matured sexually, self-pleasuring allows an adolescent a chance to learn about his or her own physiology—erection and ejaculation, or lubrication and orgasm, and to experience the entire sexual response cycle.

Fantasizing about being with a person to whom one is attracted sexually prepares one for initiating adult relationships. Combining fantasy, masturbation, and sexual pleasure allows the adolescent to "practice" for a wished-for sexual encounter, integrate him or herself as a sexual being, and begin to feel more sexually competent.

Whether you fantasized or masturbated (or both) in adolescence and how you felt about it if you did had more of an impact on your sexuality than you may be aware of. Masturbation and fantasy are normal, natural activities, which, at their best, have many benefits for sexual development and self-growth.

However, some young boys and girls who grow up in an unempathic family discover the powerful link between consoling themselves and sexual pleasure. Then, when they're really angry and feel hurt and unloved by their parents, they masturbate to feel better. When there is an ongoing struggle between parent and child, the fantasies during masturbation can focus on control, dominance, or revenge. In addition, masturbation may be used compulsively to overcome feelings of emptiness. In these instances, masturbation and fantasy can interfere with your ability to have a healthy sexual relationship.

Whether or not *you* masturbated in adolescence, most of your peers did. Teenage girls are statistically less likely to masturbate than boys, but many do. In one study (Hunt 1974) one-third of the female respondents and two-thirds of the males reported having masturbated by the age of thirteen. Even now, with all the focus on teenagers having intercourse, masturbation still is probably the most commonly occurring sexual activity among adolescents. Sexual and/or romantic fantasies about peers, teachers, siblings, and others are common among adolescents, regardless of gender.

At its best, in the context of a loving, permission-giving family environment, masturbation and fantasy (without guilty feelings) can play an important role in enhancing an adolescent's sense of him- or herself as an increasingly competent, mature, sexual adult (see chapter 10 for more about adolescence). Masturbation, as well as fantasy, can be practice for pleasurable future sexual encounters.

> *I had feelings in my vagina when I was a teenager, but I wasn't sexually active yet. I didn't know how to masturbate. I tried touching myself with my fingers, which didn't do much. I tried using a carrot! That felt sort of good, but too weird. It wasn't until much later that I did some reading and learned about vibrators. That worked great. I felt a real sense of accomplishment when I could give myself an orgasm.*
>
> —Adele, 30

Boys and Masturbation

Many boys from all kinds of families discover their penis and the pleasure it can bring at a young age. Masturbation can be a way of exploring one's body and coming to terms with changes in how the body functions. It can be a way of assuring oneself that sexual urges are normal and natural. Boys are likely to make this explicitly sexual exploration a social experience in a way that girls don't.

> *I have great memories of the time I spent hanging around with the boys in the neighborhood. We had a lot of fun together, and they taught me all about sexuality. Boy, we were really girl crazy. We just loved girls.*
>
> *I was one of the youngest ones in the group. They kind of initiated me. They showed me how to masturbate. I had never done it. One guy had a whole stack of girlie magazines, and we used to masturbate with them. We used to talk about making love to girls. It was funny, we used to believe that if you knew just the right way to touch a girl, she would just go crazy for you. I look back on these memories quite fondly.*
>
> —Craig, 47

As sociologist John Gagnon commented (1972, 239), "These secret meetings engender guilt and anxiety, but at the same time, by publicly and socially acting out their newfound sexuality, the boys cement their own sense of themselves as sexual beings, and help each other through what often are sad feelings at the emotional separation from childhood and their parents. These male-male discussions and comparisons serve to regularize and order and further motivate the sexual behavior."

Girls and Masturbation

For girls, guilt-free masturbation and fantasy also are healthy, solidifying their sense of themselves as sexual beings, giving them self-confidence, and teaching them about their bodies:

> *I remember, at about age six or so, learning how to masturbate for the first time. I was playing around in the tub, and discovered that if I ran water over my vulva, I got all kinds of good feelings. As I got older, I*

experimented more and more with the water in the tub, and then I learned that I could give myself an orgasm with my fingers. That freed me up from the bathtub, and gave me many, many hours of nighttime pleasure in my bed. By the time I was an adolescent, I could give myself really strong orgasms. I thought it was a pretty neat trick!

Actually, the first time I had intercourse with a boy, at eighteen, my first year in college, I was surprised that the experience was not nearly as satisfying as what I could do for myself! I finally figured out, and pretty quickly at that, that I better teach my boyfriend how I like to be touched. Then, I really liked intercourse.

Another big benefit of my great skill at masturbation was that I was able to use it to lessen my sexual tensions, especially in between boyfriends.

—Sandra, 38

Sandra's experience was wonderfully liberating, sexually. Clearly, she benefited by being in charge of her own sexual pleasure. She also incorporated a new sense of herself into her body image, and initiated herself, at her own pace, into sexual adulthood. Sandra's situation as a girl isn't all that common. If you had a similar experience, you were lucky, indeed.

In most cultures about which we have information, masturbation is more common among boys than among girls. And although many girls masturbate in adolescence, the context is very different than among boys. There is no huge upsurge in sexual behavior during girls' adolescence, and no group sexual behavior which legitimizes and socializes it.

Parents are much more protective of girls. Sociologist John Gagnon comments that instead of getting socialized to become sexual beings, girls are trained in "docility." What they are taught about menstruation is tied to reproduction, not sexuality. And the discussions, reinforced by peers and parents alike, are about love, romance, and marriage. Unless a girl has been hypersexualized by sexual abuse, or an overly sexualized family environment, fantasies are more likely to be romantic and vague, rather than genital.

I didn't date in high school, and I don't remember having any sexual fantasies. I didn't even consider masturbating. The sense of myself that I got from my father and brother teasing me convinced me that no one would want me, sexually or in any other way. I don't think I believed that I was attractive until my late twenties, and it was only then that I really explored masturbation and sexual relationships with others.

—Selena, age 56

Problems with Masturbation

Guilt

For children and adolescents to learn about their sexuality, they need permission, as well as freedom of time and space, to masturbate. We have seen that at its best, masturbating provides a way to "practice" having intercourse. It can lead to feelings of pleasure and competence. But, if the child is raised in a very negative sexual environment, masturbation can lead to guilt, depression, self-disgust, or self-labeling as immature and perverted.

I was told that masturbation was"bad" for people physically and emotionally

—Sherry, 43

In adolescence, at fourteen or fifteen, I was caught experimenting sexually with a same sex friend. I was not spoken to for a month. I felt terribly ashamed, alone and isolated. I still tend to feel that sexual expression is something to be ashamed about and that it must be done in great secrecy.

—Tim, 26

For a long time, I felt masturbation was a childlike thing, which left me feeling guilty.

—Greg, 30

John came from a family that didn't touch affectionately at all and who thought sex was dirty. What he learned in his family was to split people into two camps: the "good" people, who weren't sexual, and the "nasty" people, who were. As an adult, of course he wanted to be able to enjoy sex, but he had a tough time. He had a lot of trouble picturing himself as a "sexy" person. When he would make love to his wife, Jenny, if he began to lose his erection, he couldn't use fantasy to arouse himself because he had no sexual fantasies.

As it turns out, he had not masturbated as an adolescent at all—not in private, and not in groups. Besides the family prohibition on masturbation, there was no place to go to be alone! The house was small and he lived in an attic alcove that had no door. The only safe place to be alone was in the shower, and even then, his mother walked in and took things out of the medicine closet while he was in the shower. Because he didn't have permission, or any place, or any way to practice being sexual, his sexual identity remained tentative and childlike.

In adult men, an inability to be successful with erections and intercourse sometimes turns out to be tied to a history of having been inhibited from masturbating as an adolescent. In most cases, it isn't the lack of masturbating, *alone*, which causes the problem. But when a lack of experience masturbating combines with an earlier block in sexual unfolding, such as an absence of touch, a poor body image, a sex-negative family, or poor social skills, sexual development can get derailed.

Lance suffered lifelong erectile difficulties, caused by a series of developmental factors, including lack of permission, body image problems, and an adolescent fear of masturbation. He grew up in the Texas Bible Belt, in a family of hard-working factory workers. Lance married Susan a year ago. They began sex therapy because Lance had never been successful at having an erection, and they had never completed intercourse. Susan was in a lot of distress and felt that she was not sure she could stay married to Lance, much as she loved him, if his sexual difficulties weren't solved.

As his history unfolded in sex therapy, it became clear what had happened. Lance had been a shy boy, and very overweight. His parents were loving, but they firmly believed that most aspects of sexuality were sinful, including masturbation and premarital sex. Lance revered them, and he took their attitudes to heart.

As a young boy, he always felt shy and defective about his weight. He was teased about it in school, and he grew to feel ashamed of his body.

When he was about ten, he had some experiences running around with a group of older boys, and listening to them talk about masturbating. They didn't feel bad or sinful about it, and they described and illustrated ejaculating. Lance was younger and not sexually mature yet, but he was curious.

He went home, and guiltily, he tried to masturbate. He found the experience upsetting. He felt dirty, didn't experience touching his penis as pleasurable, couldn't fantasize, and since he wasn't sexually mature yet, it "didn't work" (he couldn't ejaculate). Furthermore, masturbating made him focus on his defective body image, which made him more anxious.

He tried masturbating a few more furtive times, after he got older, also without enjoying it. He had mild anxiety that something was "wrong with him" sexually, but he convinced himself that when he finally was ready to meet the right girl and get married, everything would be fine. He gave up on masturbation and fantasy.

In agricultural college, at nineteen, he got serious with a girl. He felt so committed to her that he no longer felt it would be sinful to be sexual. He was okay with kissing and touching, but when it was time to have intercourse, he was so frightened that he couldn't get an erection. Now, he became really worried. What was wrong with him?

A year later, he met Susan. The performance problems persisted, and they entered sex therapy.

Lance finally became potent, after almost two years of sex therapy focusing on his guilt about masturbating, the tie-in to his body image, and activities designed to help him to enjoy fantasizing and masturbating.

Ron came into sex therapy, referred by a urologist, complaining of an inability to ejaculate with his girlfriend. Ron wouldn't masturbate at all, and he had terrible nonspecific prostatitis, as a result. Gender identification problems and disgust with masturbation seemed to be major contributors to his physical and psychological problems.

Ron had grown up with his brother, raised by his mother in a single-parent household. Ron's father had deserted his mother for another woman when Ron was nine. Ron has vivid memories of his mother, depressed and crying, when his father left. The father moved to another state, and stayed in loose contact with his two children.

Ron loved his mother very much, and was grateful to her for being such an attentive, concerned parent. As a kid, he felt understood by her and liked to talk to her for hours and hours. He had nothing good to say about his father.

Looking at Ron's past, a number of things became apparent. First, a major dynamic was Ron's disgust at the normal sexual behavior of his own gender. He thought that men were "idiots, ruled by their cocks and their sexual passions . . . they take what they want and then leave." Because he felt so strongly about men being aggressive and treating women as sexual objects, Ron refused to masturbate and fantasize as an adolescent.

Even when told that masturbation would probably cure his prostatitis, Ron refused to masturbate. He hated using fantasy materials to get aroused, and his feelings of disgust were so strong that he felt no pleasure during masturbation.

Ron was an ardent feminist who believed that men took advantage of women, and he had very strong moral ideas about what kinds of sexual behavior were permissible between men and women. He spent a lot of time talking with his girlfriend, paying attention to her thoughts and feelings. The other issue contributing to his inability to ejaculate with his girlfriend was his fear of eventually hurting her. He wasn't sure that he would marry her. Unconsciously, he equated intercourse and ejaculation with a major commitment. Ron didn't want to be a "jerk" like his father, who he felt had used women and then thrown them away. He was acting out his fear of hurting his girlfriend by withholding his semen.

Evolution may have planned the urge to masturbate on purpose. Apes do it, dogs and cats do it, elephants do it, and even porcupines do it. Boys and men may be programmed to do it in an effort to increase fertility, because new sperm are formed continuously.

Storing seminal fluids for long periods can cause prostate congestion, which can then lead to urinary or ejaculatory distress. Regular ejaculation, either through masturbation or intercourse, can help ward off the kind of prostatitis that Ron had (which is also called "priest's disease" or "sailor's disease.")

Bart was another adult whose adulthood sexual problems stemmed from issues where blocks about masturbating combined with prior developmental obstacles. Bart's parents' poor marital relationship interfered with his sexual identity as a man. Bart had never been successful keeping his erection during intercourse, and came into sex therapy with his girlfriend as a result.

Bart grew up, one of two children, in an unhappy home. He loved his mother, but hated his father. His father treated his mother quite badly. The father was physically abusive toward her on a number of occasions, and Bart tried to intervene and stop him.

Bart's mother turned to him for companionship and compassion. She took him with her everywhere, and told him all of her problems. She also was incredibly intrusive.

When Bart was an adolescent, she actively interfered in his masturbating. Bart's bed had a wooden headboard and was placed next to a wall. If his mother heard his bed rattling around, she would come in and tell him to "stop thrashing around and go to bed." She also came into the bedroom to "check him" at night, supposedly because she wanted to make sure that her teenaged son was properly covered with the blankets—Bart got the clear message that he was not supposed to masturbate.

At the same time, like Ron, Bart felt a lot of self-hate at becoming a man. He couldn't allow himself to fantasize about being sexual with a woman because he didn't feel good about relationships between the sexes.

Bart didn't have many experiences with women as a teenager. Because he didn't feel good about leaving home and leaving his mother alone in the house with his abusive father, Bart commuted to college from home his first year.

Although he left home and went away to college the next year, being sexual with women didn't feel comfortable or familiar to him. The first time he actually tried to have intercourse, he couldn't get an erection. This set up a pattern of performance anxiety that persisted until he sought treatment, over twenty years later.

One of the changes in adolescence (see chapter 10) is a newfound ability to think abstractly and symbolically. Moral categories and oppositions (good and evil, purity and degradation) and gender role activities (aggression and submission, control and freedom) can become attached to masturbating. In the examples of Bart and Ron, the boys' family histories and disturbed gender identifications invested masturbation with special, upsetting meanings.

Objectification

Most adolescent boys don't worry about the "politics" of the fantasies they are using when they masturbate. In early adolescence, many sexual fantasies, especially for boys, are of desired "sex objects"—not real people with their own needs and desires. But if your early rearing was empathetic and power was handled well, at your core, you believe it is safe to trust and love. As you mature into an older adolescent, you begin to integrate your sexual urges and desires and fantasies with a wish to be emotionally close to your partner.

However, if your parents were emotionally absent, or harsh and unsupportive, then your adolescent masturbation fantasies might have involved a script about being in control or getting revenge on women, and you might never mature to a stage where you want to be both sexually and emotionally close to another person.

> Martin came from a family that was unempathic and distant, and even in his twenties, the way he talks about his dates with women, clearly indicates that he doesn't really see women as whole people—just bodies and sexual organs to be conquered:

> "Well, I was hoping that you could help me get my erection back sooner than it comes back these days. I'm dating a couple of girls now, and it's really great, you know, having all that sex. This one girl, she's really pretty. And she gives me oral sex, which is great. So I go out with her a lot. But I like to see a couple of girls over the weekend, and have sex. But, I'm upset, because if I had sex a couple of times on Friday with one girl, then sometimes on Saturday, I can't even get it up with the next girl. And that's not right. I'm only twenty-two. What can I do so that I can have sex a couple of times each night?"

Male Masturbation: Helpful or Hurtful?

What goes on in boys' secret society of masturbation may be "predatory" by today's politically correct standards. Yet, some amount of "objectifying" women in fantasies may well be a necessary component of heterosexual male sexual development. As we sex therapists see fairly frequently, adult males who are afraid of hurting their partner with their erect penises have difficulty performing the sexual act. The masturbation-group's socially sanctioned, acted out aggressive performances may help them get over this fear.

Among heterosexual men, someone like Martin has had too much practice objectifying women, and not enough empathy and attachment to the real women in his life. He uses women sexually and can't connect to them emotionally. It's likely that even if he "falls in love" and marries at some point, his sexual arousal might be more tied to how his partner looks than to any deep feelings he might have about her.

On the other hand, Bart and Ron have the opposite problem. They were deeply scarred by their father's selfish behavior. They are over-identified with their mothers, unseparated, and literally disgusted by their own gender because of the way their fathers acted. Bart and Ron are so fearful of male aggression and genital sexuality, that they can't let themselves feel lust. Their lack of practicing masculine, genital sexuality—through fantasy and masturbation—in adolescence led to anxiety and performance problems with women later on.

Guilt-free masturbation, in John's case, would have helped him have a better marital relationship. Between his parents' sex-evasive and sex negative attitudes and the lack of affection in his family, his sexual growth was stunted.

Early adolescent boys' fantasies aren't necessarily adult fantasies; the women aren't fully human. They are just sex toys. But if the pre-adolescent environment is a caring, trusting one, with healthy gender identity models, if the boys aren't controlled or punished harshly, and if their social skills are good enough—then, later in adolescence, they will be able to combine masturbation and sexual fantasies with images of love. They will be able to make the switch to real whole-person relationships with young women.

Compulsive Masturbation

Occasionally soothing yourself with masturbation can be a normal part of sexual development. However, when adolescent boys and girls chronically use masturbation to get away from the frustration and emotional pain of living in an abusive, authoritarian family, problems can result. Masturbation to orgasm does provide a physical release, and the behavior is reinforced. This can lead to a lifelong pattern of sexual compulsion. All pain is dealt with through sexual release.

I was so frustrated on that long drive home from work, and so angry that Jane doesn't keep the house clean or make a nice dinner for me, that before I knew what was happening, I found myself in the combat zone, getting a blow job from a hooker.

I honestly don't know how I got there. It's like I was on automatic pilot. But then, you know, I think, "Well, I worked hard all day. I deserved that."

—Sean, 33

Sexual Addiction

When the family environment contains only disappointment and abuse, offset with little love and empathy, sexual trouble looms. People who grow up in families which are abusive start to think that they are basically unworthy people. They also begin to believe that their needs will never be met if they have to depend on others.

As Patrick Carnes, Ph.D., points out (1992), good parenting includes touching, loving, affirming, and guiding. The child in this kind of family feels cared for even when struggling with rules and limits.

But when a child's exploration of sexuality passes self discovery to become a routine way of self-comforting, because the parents aren't emotionally available, there is potential for addiction. Sex is confused with consoling, and to feel secure means to be sexual.

Masturbation may be used as a compulsive, self-soothing mechanism during times of distress, with poor consequences for their sexual and personal development.

"Consequently, the child's relationship with people has the potential of being replaced with an addictive relationship with sexuality. Addiction is a relationship—a pathological relationship in which sexual obsession replaces people. And it can start very early. The . . . core belief of the addict emerges clearly: *Sex is my most important need.*" (pp. 71–72)

> Sean's compulsive use of masturbation to soothe his feelings of being abused led to sexual addiction and criminal activities. He came into therapy for help with his rage in his relationship with his wife. Sean was bright, funny, and charming, but he had a darker side in his family.
>
> Sean felt overworked and underappreciated, and he was exhausted by his role as the breadwinner for his wife and two small children. Sean had the capacity to love, but he had a long-smoldering rage and a difficulty with impulse control.
>
> As his trust grew, Sean revealed that he was a sexual addict. Unbeknownst to his wife, he had been seeing prostitutes and exposing himself while masturbating on his ride home. He also had exposed himself to a neighbor twice, and had gotten caught.
>
> Sean grew up in what looked like a nice, middle-class home. However, his father was a tyrant, and his mother did not protect him. His father was verbally and physically abusive, and was hypercritical of everything that Sean did.

Sean became aware of his own sexual impulse quite young, around age seven. He began masturbating, alone in his room, beginning then. As he got older, around age ten, he began to have occasional intercourse with a thirteen-year-old girl who lived nearby.

Sean used sexuality to propel himself out of the pain of his home life. As he got to be an adolescent, Sean's father only increased his dominion over him. One summer, he made Sean hand-dig a huge, deep hole for the foundation of an addition to the house. The more power Sean's father exerted, the more adolescent Sean retreated to his room, to compulsively masturbate while thinking vengeful thoughts. This set the pattern for the way Sean thinks about his sexual desires—as his just reward during tough times.

Besides visiting prostitutes, Sean also exposed himself. Sean's activity exposing himself is a criminal offense, but he never went so far as to physically and aggressively touch or hurt another person. He did have the capacity to connect to his wife and children, and he got real pleasure out of his relationship with them. As his therapy uncovered what had gone wrong in his family, his sexual compulsions improved. If you have a sexual pattern like Sean's, get professional help, because you can change.

Anna grew up in a filthy, chaotic home. Her father went off to work each day, ignoring the fact that his wife was a terrible alcoholic who physically abused and neglected Anna and her sister, Tiesha. Anna's pediatrician never seemed to pick up on the fact that Anna had an unusual number of sprains and twice had a broken arm. There wasn't much relief from the insecurity and the maltreatment.

Anna discovered masturbation when she was about seven, when she found out that if she squeezed her favorite teddy bear between her legs, she got nice feelings. Whenever her mother hurt her or hit her, she began masturbating compulsively, but secretly. It felt good to her to take care of her own needs.

She didn't have many friends, but she began to act out sexual fantasies on Tiesha, who was four years younger. Anna made Tiesha perform sexual acts on her, and swore her to silence. She began a pattern of penetrating Tiesha with her finger, and was obsessed with fantasies involving rape.

After she left her family, Anna felt scared and lonely. She felt ashamed of what she had done with Tiesha and swore that she would never abuse anyone else again.

Anna didn't continue to abuse others, but she continued to abuse herself. She didn't really trust anyone, man or woman alike. She had no idea how to form a friendship or a relationship. She didn't even really like men.

But when she felt empty, she couldn't stand the feelings, and she felt compelled to seek out a sexual partner. She went to bars, and had hundreds of one-night stands with men over the course of three years. It was a temporary sexual fix, and she remained as lonely as ever. It was only when she got very sick, and confronted an AIDS scare, that she stopped and looked at the fact that her life was out of control and that she was a sex addict.

Sexual Predators

At the most extreme, in very violent families, the feelings associated with adult relationships may well elicit too much fear and anger to be associated with sexual arousal, and the child may learn to masturbate and get sexually aroused imagining something safe: an object, other children, sexual deviations such as getting sexual pleasure by watching others. As the child enters puberty, these fantasies persist. Then the fantasies are linked to the pleasure of arousal and this behavior is reinforced by the physical release orgasm brings. The responses become conditioned to various stressful or sexual situations.

In the worst case scenario, masturbation to sadistic scripts in adolescence and adulthood can help create coercive sexual predators and criminals: Boys (and girls) who grew up in violent, controlling environments may learn to tie arousal and orgasm to sadistic, masochistic, or forcible fantasies. Orgasms are a powerful reinforcer of the sadistic fantasies. Eventually these acts may actually be carried out. The recidivism rate among aggressive sex criminals is quite high.

Learning Now What You Didn't Learn Then

Most American adults grew up in reasonably good families and aren't in danger of becoming sexual sadists. Most Americans, men and women alike, are more likely to have been hampered sexually by a historic lack of permission to explore their bodies, fantasize, and masturbate. If this describes your experience, learning to masturbate and fantasize can be an important step in reaching your sexual potential.

Typically, adults who have been inhibited can overcome their fears about masturbation. They begin to successfully use self-pleasuring to find out what their sexual likes and dislikes are.

> Betsy, who at thirty-five lives with her mother for economic reasons, needed to experiment with sexual pleasure and orgasms in order to be more orgasmic with her boyfriend—but she had a lot of obstacles to overcome before she became competent at masturbation.
>
> Her mother actually was very open to all of this, but Betsy somehow felt too shy to ask for privacy. It was a small house, and the laundry room, where her mother not only did washing, but quite a bit of ironing, was down the hall from her room. Even if Betsy took a long time to get into the mood and lie there, her concentration was broken by hearing her mother walk back and forth to the ironing board.
>
> In addition, she had a difficult time stimulating herself with her hand, but felt using a vibrator was too mechanical and she couldn't let herself enjoy it. She was concerned with the noise the vibrator made, and couldn't relax and let herself fantasize because she felt too uptight with her mother in the same house.
>
> After quite a long time brainstorming, Betsy took a huge risk. She asked her mother to give her a few hours in the house alone on Saturdays. Her mother agreed, and Betsy began to experiment with using the vibrator. As she got more comfortable, she learned that it was okay to masturbate with the vibrator when her mother was in the house, as long as she put loud music on the stereo. As she learned what she liked, physically, her sexual relationship with her boyfriend improved.

If you haven't masturbated before now, it takes a while to get used to the feelings, and it takes time to label the feelings you do feel as pleasure. Be patient. Be creative. Several excellent books, listed in the Resources section for this chapter, will help you.

Exercises

Assess Your Feelings About Masturbation

Read the following lists of feelings (positive, neutral, and negative) about masturbation. Circle all that apply to your experiences.

Positive feelings about masturbation:

- I feel fine about it. Masturbation is a natural activity that normal people use throughout life.

- I used it to reduce tension in a healthy way.

- I used it to visualize sexual encounters that I wanted to have with real people. I think it was helpful.

- I think I used it to understand and integrate my own sexuality.

Neutral feelings about masturbation and fantasy:

- I didn't masturbate or fantasize, and I think it was okay.

- I did masturbate or fantasize, and I think it was okay.

Negative feelings about masturbation or fantasy:

- I didn't masturbate or fantasize. In looking back, I feel my family environment was too restrictive.

- I wish I had been able to use masturbation or fantasy in a positive way, but I wasn't able to. I think it might have helped me in these ways:

_____

_____

_____

- I did it, but I felt really guilty about it.

- I used masturbation to avoid interactions with my peers; I think it was used in a bad way, as an escape.

- The fact that I used masturbation as much as I did makes me feel that I am sexually inept.

- I used it to soothe myself in a somewhat compulsive way. (If so, what feelings were you trying to avoid having?)

_____

_____

_____

Identifying Your Central Masturbation Fantasy.

Did you have a central or main masturbation fantasy? What was it? Did it change over time? Do you still use it now?

_____

_____

_____

Are You Sexually Compulsive?

Answer the following questions.

	Yes	No
• There was violence in my family of origin.	____	____
• On some level, I don't really trust people.	____	____
• I basically assume I have to meet all of my own needs.	____	____
• I learned to use sexuality and masturbation to soothe myself when things got too tough to stand in my family.	____	____
• I consciously use sexuality when life is hard.	____	____
• There are times when I automatically use sexual behaviors when I am upset, rather than using other techniques to calm down.	____	____
• I don't feel able to stop masturbating or using other compulsive sexual behavior.	____	____
• I sometimes worry that I have used other people sexually in a manipulative way.	____	____

If you answered yes to the first question, be sure to read chapter 11 on violence in this book for more exercises.

If you answered yes to more than four of the above questions, the negative power dynamics in your family have *clearly* contributed to your sexual difficulty. Either you are unable to use sexuality in order to express a deep connection to another person, or you are using sexuality (including masturbation and fantasy) in an addictive or abusive fashion.

Are You a Sex Addict?

If you have a problem using sex in an addictive way, make an inventory of the ways you have used sexuality to control or hurt others. Make the list historically, by date, starting at the beginning of the pattern. Use a separate piece of paper or your journal if you need more room for this exercise.

You may be using sexuality for stress-control instead of for connecting to other people. Sexuality can block painful feelings, because an orgasm has a great capacity to reduce tension. Begin keeping a journal of your daily experiences with using sexuality (including masturbation) as a way of soothing yourself. Keep track of when you used a compulsive sexual activity, what feeling you believe you were avoiding, and what other kind of stress-relieving activity you could have used in its place.

Date	Time	Upsetting Event	Type of Compulsive Activity	Avoided Feeling	Alternative Action You Could Have Taken

If you feel you have a compulsive sexual addiction, there are a lot of relatively new sources of help available, as well. See the Resources section at the end of this book.

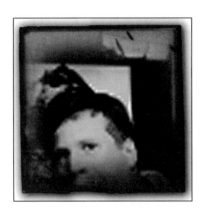

Chapter 10

The Changes of Adolescence

Adolescents everywhere experience intense sexual curiosity and desire.
—Leonore Tiefer, *Human Sexuality: Feelings and Functions*

♦ What was adolescence like for you?

♦ How do you feel about the way you transited it?

♦ When you think about your adolescence, do you feel ashamed, pleased, angry?

♦ How did you express your sexuality as an adolescent?

♦ Was your sexuality harmed by unwanted or unfortunate experiences in adolescence? If so, how has your sexuality been affected?

♦ Did you have intercourse as an adolescent? If so, were your sexual relationships with peers, or were you seduced by a person who was older?

♦ Was your sexual experience in the context of a genuine, deep, ongoing relationship with mutual empathy?

♦ Did you use birth control/prophylactics?

♦ Did you feel in charge of your sexuality?

♦ If you are bisexual or homosexual, when and how did you first figure out your sexual orientation? How did you feel about this realization? If you told your parents during your adolescence, how they did react?

A Transformation

Adolescence is a time of great change. Even if your family did a fine job of creating a nurturing environment, helping you to feel good about yourself, handling power, providing you with appropriate knowledge of sexuality, and encouraging your social skills, you may have floundered anew during the special strains of adolescence. Adolescence is a pivotal stage in a child's development, when several tasks must be accomplished before entering adulthood.

As an adolescent, you needed to come to terms with your changing body and your changing sexual urges. You had to separate emotionally from your family of origin, establishing autonomy as well as fitting in with your peer group. Adolescence is a time of exploration, when sexual behavior, both self-stimulation and partnered, generally increases. Over the last four decades, there has been an increase in the number of adolescents who have experienced intercourse, although almost a third of adolescents have not had sexual intercourse by the age of nineteen.

If your adolescent sexuality was wildly destructive or distorted, then the factors underlying the psychological, social, and sexual wreckage began earlier. Problems with trust, empathy, control, guilt, and/or gender identity—to name just a few—began well before your teenage years. Emotionally neglectful families tend to totally abandon adolescents, as if they are old enough to be on their own entirely, and can cause the adolescent to withdraw, becoming even more socially isolated. Other neglected adolescents tend to act out sexually, in an attempt to get love and attention they are deprived of at home.

> *During adolescence, I was out in left field. My parents' criticism, and my general low self-esteem, and the way I felt about how I looked made it too frightening to try to get in with any of the crowds at school. I just retreated into fixing cars and riding my motorcycle. It took me until my second year of high school to come out of my shell. A girl named Gaby liked me, and she included me with her friends. I finally found out what I had been missing.*
>
> —Kyle, 27

Any less-than-ideal family sexual environments (as described in chapter 7) greatly impacts a child's adolescence, and can impair their sexual development into adulthood. Negative environments, where sexuality was seen as dirty, can create guilt and fear and difficulty coming to terms with surging sexual impulses and integrating them into one's sense of self. Seductive and overtly abusive sexual environments overencourage and over-stimulate sexuality, which can lead to feelings of disgust about sexuality in adulthood.

> *When I look back at it, my mother was just off the wall in the way she reacted to my adolescence. It was like she was in some kind of sexual competition with me. She started talking about sex all the time. It gave me the creeps, actually. It went way past what would have been a healthy, open discussion about sexuality. I felt like she was prying into my sex life, to get off sexually herself. She just wouldn't leave me alone!!*
>
> —Annie, 29

Your Changing Body

Do you remember the feelings with which you greeted the emergence of your first pubic hair, first ejaculation, or first menstrual period? Had you been prepared in advance for these occurrences? Do you remember the way your family reacted to the normal changes in your body?

Girls mature an average of two years before boys, and parents frequently are caught off guard by their daughter's sexual development. Most boys have their first ejaculation between twelve and thirteen, usually from masturbation or sexual dreams at night. The same hormonal changes that stimulate the physical development from child to adult also bring other normal changes: intensified sexual feelings and fantasies, more frequent spontaneous erections, increased vaginal lubrication, and a higher incidence of masturbation.

These changes in your body had social significance, because adolescence is the time when society at large, your parents, peers, the schools, and the media recognized your sexual capacities. Sociologist John Gagnon, Ph.D. (1972), emphasizes that to some extent, the sexualization of adolescence is invented—a social construction. The truth is, even though the capacity for orgasm (as separate from ejaculation in males) is available to younger children, there is no sense in which society recognizes this sexual capacity in preadolescent children.

In early adolescence, social and sexual development at times seems quite uncoordinated. It is possible for young boys to still be playing tag and using *Playboy* to masturbate, and for girls to still be playing with Barbie dolls or take stuffed animals to bed as they are also talking about boys.

Sometimes the meanings of the physical changes are more important than the changes themselves.

Undoubtedly, though, the physical changes that mark the beginning of adolescence are quite variable. Developing much faster, or slower, than your peers can be a terrible source of embarrassment or shame.

> *I was growing up in this tiny school in rural Utah. I already felt different. I was the smartest girl in the whole school. I had no friends. And to make matters even worse, when I was twelve, I grew these really* huge *breasts, I was a 32D. The boys wouldn't leave me alone. They snapped my bra everywhere, in the hallways, in classes. I couldn't escape. To this day, I am paranoid about passing strange men, and do the best I can to camouflage my body.*
>
> —Barbara, 35

> *I absolutely hated to go to gym in the ninth grade. I was still so short, and I hadn't developed at all. I hardly had any pubic hair, and I didn't have muscles, and my penis was tiny. And there was a group of boys who, I swear, were seven or eight inches taller than me, and fully developed. It was torture. They laughed and made snickering comments in front of me and behind my back.*
>
> *I had a growth spurt when I was in college, and I wound up to be five feet eleven inches tall, but in my mind, I'm still back in ninth grade. My body image is of a tiny, skinny boy. I still feel vulnerable in group showers.*
>
> —Tom, 26

The reactions of your parents to these physical changes had a big role to play in how you felt about them yourself. Those responses depended on the rules of their subcultural and ethnic group, and also on your parent's feelings about their own lives and their sexuality.

Obviously, families which had provided ideal, open environments for the discussion of sexuality all along would be likely to handle the adolescent issues well. But these families tend to be in the minority in the United States.

> *During my teenage years, I was never given any information about sex, nor permission to ask. This left me wondering what was normal, right, and appropriate.*
>
> —Blair, 36

When I was twelve and thirteen, my father was overly concerned about my sexuality and had exaggerated fears about my behavior with boys. I felt some sense of guilt in dating, and also a wish to act out for revenge.

—Bobbie, 35

My father would say negative things about women who dressed in an overtly sexual way—a great deal of makeup, short skirt, tight pants, a revealing or low-cut blouse. Mostly, he commented about strangers, but occasionally about my mother or myself. It made me believe that a woman looking sexual was wrong, bad, and shameful.

—Jan, 29

I had a lot of confusion over what is acceptable, what is respectful. I gained weight to be less sexually provocative.

—Alma, 46

Parents' Reactions to Girls

Far too many teenage girls are absolutely ignorant about their own bodies and have no interactions with their mothers with regard to explicit instructions about their sexual organs. Often, in childhood, boys and their dads stand side by side, each holding their penis to urinate—permission to touch is taken for granted. Girls and their moms, however, don't have any parallel interaction. This is quite unfortunate, and can hinder a girl's understanding of her own anatomy as well as her learning to feel comfortable touching herself and being touched by others (whether it be during a routine gynecological exam or during her sexual encounters).

My mother is very modest. She never taught me anything about my body. She could never even stand to talk to me about my period, and she never talked to me about tampons.

Needless to say, when I went alone to a gynecologist to get some birth control, I was totally unprepared for the whole ordeal. I had no idea that I was going to have to get up on that table, in a position like that. And I got really scared when I saw the speculum. I had no idea that they were going to put it into me. I was really frightened.

—Sarah, 23

Mothers respond to the start of menstruation in vastly different ways. One mother slapped her daughter across the face. Her daughter found out, later, that this was an old Italian custom, but at forty-nine, it still brings tears to her eyes when she thinks about it. Another mother proudly asked the daughter if she could tell the father (the daughter said no), and then took her out to a special lunch to celebrate. Yet another mother chose that moment to make a big deal out of how important it was to wash the blood stains out of your panties right away, and gave her daughter a washing lesson that very instant. And still another responded with a searing lecture about premarital sex.

> *Once I got my period, my mother seems to have gotten frantic about the possibility that I would get in trouble, even though I was impossibly shy. She would make me frightened of any kind of social contact with boys. She would say things like, "Sylvia was sitting on boys' laps. And you know what THAT means. And Joanna stayed out too late with her boyfriend, and you know what THAT means . . ." She made me so frightened of my own sexuality that I wasn't even able to enjoy kissing a boy, all the way through high school.*
>
> —Benita, 40

A teenager's budding sexuality affects the parents' feelings about themselves and each other. Ideally, the parents react with pride and joy to watching their children at the brink of adult life.

Joe remarked at how beautiful, and how sexual, his daughter looked:

"Wow, I look up, and here is my little baby girl, Jennifer, going out to a party, in a dress. And, I mean, she's a knockout. And she has no *idea*. She has no idea how she looks, no idea how much she has changed, no idea how men will respond to her. I feel like, boy, I've got to pay attention to what I'm thinking and feeling. And Jennifer still likes to come over and sit on my lap, like old times. I guess I'll have to find some way to tell her she is getting a little too old to sit on my lap. . . ."

Joe, being a father who has a lot of insight, responds to his daughter's budding beauty and sexuality, and his own sexual attraction, by complimenting her on how gorgeous she looks, and by taking note of his own sexual feelings. In addition, he shared his emotions about the transformation in his daughter with his wife, with whom he is close.

At sixteen, Francesca was getting ready to go on a summer vacation with the family. She had just gone out shopping with her best friend and had bought herself a very tricky two piece bathing suit. It was an unusual color, brown and white checks. And although the suit was not teeny and covered her completely, it was daring in that the top sections covering her breasts were held together with a metal loop in the middle of the chest, and the bottom half had similar metal loops on the sides keeping the front and back pieces together. The suit was stunning and would attract a lot of attention.

She tried it on for her mother. Her mother was overwhelmed with how Fran had grown up and startled at how gorgeous she looked. She told Fran that she looked great and that she should show her Dad. Dad was equally startled at what had become of his little girl, but simply opened his eyes wide, said, "Wow!" and whistled.

Many adult women have memories of their fathers or mothers, less mature and giving, or more anxious about their own sexuality, or more upset about their own lives, reacting to the girl's developing body in negative or competitive ways. "Watching their children, at the brink of adult life, with all options open to them can bring up feelings of discontent at how the parent's own lives have turned out," comments psychologist Lawrence Steinberg (1994, 91).

I had the sense that my mother was fearful of my becoming sexual and that males were bad, evil. Especially males that I didn't know and my mother didn't know. Now I sense my mother was struggling with recalling her own early sexual experiences. I still wonder what, if anything, happened to her to create this fear. One particularly upsetting event for me was her intense reaction to a boy asking me to a dance. She yelled, screamed and forbade me to go, as I feared she would—not a pleasant feeling.

—Lucille, 62

Ideally, as the child's body changes and the child becomes a young adult, parents will celebrate their burgeoning sexuality and give them good feedback about how they look, which helps to build sexual self-esteem. Unfortunately, because of societal rules about girls needing to be pretty, and the double standard of sexual behavior, a great number of adolescent girls get disturbing, harmful sexual feedback in adolescence, that can have serious repercussions in their adult sexual life.

Tabitha came into sex therapy to get over severe inhibitions which prevented her from experiencing sexual excitement. She loved her husband, and could get quite aroused. But somehow, before she actually had her orgasm, she would turn herself off.

As she was looking at her past experiences in her family, she came up with memory after memory of her father acting as if a woman with sexual feelings was a whore. When she was about ten, she recalls him looking up at her older sister, aged about eighteen, who was dressed up and getting ready to go on a date with her steady boyfriend, and muttering something about her sister being "like a damn bitch in heat."

Tina came into psychotherapy because she could not enjoy sexual relations with her husband. In fact, she had never felt comfortable being sexual with a boy, ever. Part of the problem may have been Tina's relationship with her father. He believed men should rule the roost and was controlling, and not warm at all. More importantly, however, he filled her with deep terror of men's sexuality.

Tina commented, "When I became a teenager, my father filled me with fears about being with men. He told me they would put a drug in my drink and then force me to have sex while I was defenseless."

Parents' Reaction to Boys

There is a dramatic difference in parents' reactions to their sons' emergence as sexual beings, since North American society and many parents hold a double standard. Boys don't need to be virgins at the time of marriage. Boys aren't usually raped. Boys can't become pregnant. So most mothers and fathers don't react to changes in the boys' bodies with panic.

It really makes me furious to think of the different ways that my brothers and I were treated when we hit our teenage years. When he was fifteen or sixteen, Bobby dressed like a punker and was drinking a lot and coming in the wee hours. He was going out with two different girls, and sleeping with both of them, as far as I can tell. Tommy, who was eighteen, had a steady girlfriend, and they were always necking in our TV room. Mom and Dad didn't say a thing.

But I wasn't allowed to "act cheap" or "look cheap." I couldn't wear red lipstick. There was this big fuss over my clothes, the tightness of my sweaters, the shortness of my skirts. And I had to be in by eleven o'clock, even when I was eighteen. Their rules and their overprotectiveness made me the butt of all my friends' jokes, and I feel like I lost out on some important experiences with boys that I'm trying to make up for now.

—Judy, 26

But neither do parents prepare boys or respond to the obvious changes in adolescence with the needed information.

My father was so cold that I didn't feel comfortable with him. When I had my first wet dream, I really wanted to talk to my mother. But she got embarrassed, and she blushed, and she just went in to her book shelf and got a book and gave it to me. I never asked her about anything sexual again.

—Jonathan, 57

Boys need to know that wet dreams are normal, that most boys have them, that nothing is physically wrong with them, and what to do with the messy sheets. Between ten and twelve, most boys discover the pleasures of masturbation, and parents must be comfortable talking about it. Sex educator Mary Calderone believes that when parents cannot allow their young sons to discover their bodies as a source of pleasure, these sons will be unable to find satisfaction in their adult sexual relationships.

Parents tend to minimize their adolescent children's questions about sexuality and their changing bodies. In *Raising a Child Conservatively in a Sexually Permissive World* (1983, 215–216), authors/sex educators Sal and Judith Gordon asked a group of twelve-year-old boys in an Ohio suburban school system to submit a list of questions they had about sex. Common questions were

- What is an erection?

- Is it normal to jack off?

- I haven't had any wet dreams. Why?

- What is 4 play?(sic)

- My friends talk about cum (sic). What is cum (sic)?

Most parents in North America are not comfortable answering these kinds of basic questions for their sons. (Just as they are not comfortable talking about sexual pleasure—as opposed to reproduction—with their daughters.)

However, as adults, boys from reasonably loving but sex-evasive or sex-negative families may tend to have fewer sexual inhibitions than girls from such climates. First of all, boys' sexual organs are less mysterious than girls', and boys are more likely than girls to discover and practice masturbation in childhood and adolescence, even when parents' overt or covert messages forbid it. Wet dreams and involuntary ejaculations may be frightening but they are often linked with sensations of pleasure, while girls' first experience of menstruation may link blood with pain. Finally, boys' sexual expression is more social in nature, and boys who aren't taught about wet dreams and ejaculations at home can talk about it (and practice masturbating) in groups with their friends.

Although it may not cause sexual inhibition, boys' parents' inability to talk frankly with them about sexual urges or masturbation hinders boys in another way in adolescence and adulthood, diminishing their skills in responsibly integrating sexuality into relationships. Without comfortable parent-child discussions of sexuality, boys have no model of talking or negotiating about sexual wants and needs. In addition, parents miss the opportunity to teach boys that intercourse belongs in the context of a loving relationship, and that they can use masturbation to curb their sexual urges at times when intercourse is not appropriate.

Parental Competition

Unfortunately, parents sometimes feel competitive with their children. Just as the teenagers are coming into young adulthood, physically blossoming, with dewy skin and pert breasts, or with new beards and slim, muscled bodies, parents are confronting age-related changes in their looks.

My mother adored my boyfriend, Bill. I really wonder whether she was totally out of love with my father at that point. But she was really into criticizing me. As I think back on it now, I realize that the whole time I was going out with Bill, for those three years, she was on top of me about my weight. And how fat could I have been? I've always worn a size eight.

But you know, when I get my period, and I gain a pound or two, I never feel slim enough to make love . . . and I think it goes back to my mom's comments when I was in high school. Wow. It's really pitiful to think that it didn't occur to me until my thirty-sixth birthday that she was jealous of me!

—Erin, 40

Establishing a Sense of Autonomy

Another central psychological task of early adolescence is becoming an independent person—separating emotionally from one's parents. By the time they have become twelve or thirteen, most teenagers want to control their own day-to-day lives, including activities, friends, and values.

Relationships Outside the Family

In early adolescence, as described in a previous chapter, kids begin intimate friendships outside the family based on empathy, trust, and self-disclosure. It is in this period of socialization that friends become the most important people in the teenager's social world.

Teaching teenagers about sexuality is important, and studies show that this does not contribute to promiscuity. Unfortunately, however, teaching teenagers specifically about sexuality is not sufficient, because it does not necessarily teach them about intimacy.

By middle adolescence, teenagers begin to be more sophisticated about people and to appreciate that their friends have idiosyncrasies. Adolescents turn to their friends when they are disappointed, angry, or in difficulty. They learn about the ups and downs of friendship, and how you can go to different friends with different needs. At best, they learn which friends are true friends, and which friends aren't to be trusted. Early lessons about trust, empathy, and forgiveness are learned in the family—by adolescence, the give and take of relating to peers is the major arena for learning relationship skills.

While it will probably always be true that teenage boys will be more cavalier about sexual relationships than teenaged girls, in general, adolescents who didn't have empathic relationships, good modeling, and good communication in their family of origin are more likely to get into ill-advised, shallow sexual relationships and less likely to be able to have intimate (nonsexual or sexual) relationships.

Sexual coercion with a peer can contribute to negative associations to sexuality—disgust, detachment—that can take intensive work to undo as an adult.

My mother and father were really kind of cold. I didn't feel very good at home. There weren't all that many kids my age around; we lived way out in the sticks. And in this rural area where I lived, it was common for kids to go off and drink and drive their cars really fast, and goof off. There was not much else to do.

So I got involved with this crowd of older kids, with this boy, Chuck, who I thought was cool, who had a really cool car. I felt like somebody when I went out with him. We mostly just drank. We really didn't talk. But I thought it was fun.

But then he really turned on the pressure for intercourse. I was only fifteen. The first time, he really forced me. We were out in the woods. After that, we were boyfriend and girlfriend, but I kept getting coerced into doing sexual stuff. I never really felt like it.

—Debby, 25

Early and middle adolescents who have the basic social skills, as well as parental modeling of intimacy, self-esteem, and confidence learn how powerful these peer relationships can be. They learn that close connections with peers can include enjoying each other's company, mutual trust, understanding, confiding experiences and feelings to each other, and being spontaneous in the relationship. A self-assured adolescent who realizes the depth of feeling possible with a peer is less likely to settle for a shallow sexual relationship, just to be in the in-crowd, or to avoid rejection.

Integrating Your Sexuality into Your Identity

Because of the relatively puritanical sexual socialization in American society, many adolescents need to separate emotionally from their parents in order to feel free to be sexual in healthy ways, to integrate their sexuality into their identity. Not separating from parents with very rigid sexual values can cause later sexual problems.

> Morrie grew up well-loved in a highly educated, analytical, somewhat obsessive and cautious family. Rationality was prized. He respected his parents and loved them very much. His mother was warm and concerned about him, his father was a hard worker. So when they told him he should abstain from premarital sex, he took them quite literally.
>
> An older brother, much more of a family rebel, tried to encourage him to separate from his parents and to help him feel more comfortable being sexual and "wild." But Morrie just felt that his brother was "being evil and trying to corrupt me." Morrie wanted to be the "good" kid.

Morrie did not masturbate much, and he did not have inter-course throughout college. When he finally felt he had met the person he wanted to marry, in his midtwenties, he felt it was safe to have intercourse. However, his intended was a very emotional, highly sexual young woman.

Morrie was threatened by this. He felt fearful that he wouldn't know what to do sexually. When he finally had intercourse with his fiancée, he had problems with premature ejaculation, which frustrated her.

It took him some time in sex therapy to straighten out his anxiety about sexuality. In retrospect, he felt that his brother had good intentions. He also came to see that he was really too attached to his mother. She was closer to him emotionally than she was to her own husband. Morrie wished that he hadn't been so intent on being the perfect, good son. He wished, in retrospect that he had experimented more, and paid more attention to his own sexual impulses.

In other kinds of families, more unhappy ones, difficulties separating can come out of an alliance with a parent who you feel is being victimized. If you grew up in an unhappy family, where your parents didn't treat each other well, or didn't love each other, you might have become allied with one of your parents, often the parent of the opposite sex. If the struggle to break away from this parent left you feeling guilty, and you didn't separate in adolescence, you may have had problems later, emotionally or sexually.

Hugh, who was to be married in a year, began sex therapy with his fiancée, a woman who loved him a great deal. Hugh was afraid of intercourse, and couldn't maintain an erection. Besides growing up in a sexually repressive environment, the crux of Hugh's problem actually revolved around his sexual guilt and his lack of separation from his mother.

When he was about twelve or thirteen, Hugh's mother, a very depressed woman, told him the intimate details of how she had been rejected sexually by his father. Hugh spent most of his adolescence feeling angry at his father, angry at himself for being a man, and sorry for his mother. He tried to take care of her emotionally, but nothing seemed to make her feel better.

In therapy, Hugh improved as he realized that all along, he had felt guilty for letting himself have more sexual pleasure than his mother had. As he realized that he couldn't fix his mother's life, and that his primary attachment needed to be to his wife, his erectile problems resolved.

Bisexuality and Homosexuality

Although statistics vary quite a bit, it is safe to say that at least 4 percent of American males and 2 percent of American females are exclusively homosexual. (Kinsey et al. 1948; Crooks and Baur 1993). Current research implies that there may be a biological predisposition to homosexuality, and no evidence has clearly shown that childhood or family factors are a cause (Bell 1981; Ross and Arrindell 1988).

Discovering that you are homosexual in adolescence can be a very upsetting experience, compounded by the fact that most homosexual adolescents have internalized the negative and homophobic views of American culture. Many of them have even used negative labels on other gays, calling them "queers," "dykes," "sissies," or "fags." During adolescence, in a period already fraught with changing bodies, sexuality, and changing identity, homosexual and bisexual adolescents have extra stresses and strains that can lead to isolation, low self-esteem, and suicidal feelings and attempts.

Within the last few years, more is becoming understood about developmental processes among homosexual and bisexual teenagers. One excellent review of the literature is contained in a book edited by D'Augelli and Patterson (1995).

Because males and females are socialized differently in American society, gay adolescent boys and girls take different paths in becoming aware of their homosexuality. Since teenage girls are allowed a broader range of feelings and behaviors toward other girls, if you are a lesbian, you may have experienced your emerging sexual and emotional closeness as friendship, and you may not have identified yourself as lesbian or bisexual until well into adulthood.

However, if you are a homosexual male, you probably recognized your orientation during adolescence. This is because males are socialized more narrowly, and your longing for emotional and physical contact with other males probably made it more clear to you early on that you were homosexual.

Homosexual boys tend to crystallize their sexual identity more abruptly, and to focus on sexual activity while coming out. Consistent with their different socialization, lesbian teenagers may not act sexual during adolescence, instead focusing on self-absorption and reflection.

Coming Out

If you are gay or bisexual, how did you feel when you realized your sexual orientation? Usually, when teenagers realize their homosexual leanings, they get confused, and then petrified about the future rejection and persecution which they feel lies ahead of them. With adolescence already a lonely time of leaving the family, homosexual and/or bisexual teens feel completely stranded and alone.

Once you recognized a bisexual or homosexual orientation, what factors came into play in helping you make your decisions to reveal (or not reveal) your sexual orientation to others? Did you believe that you were the only gay teen in your peer group, or in your school?

Homosexual or bisexual teens may simply stay hidden, cut off from the social groups of straight kids. Or, in urban areas, in what may be a more harmful move, they may be drawn to bars and clubs, where they meet older gays and leave themselves open for exploitation.

Fear of parental disapproval among teens is so great that many hide their sexuality, both to save themselves from rejection by parents and to protect their parents from the hurt they are sure will be caused by the revelation. But this makes forming a sense of identity problematic, since they are, in essence, leading double lives. If you are homosexual or bisexual, you may have missed out on a normal rite of straight passage: having your parents meet your boyfriend or girlfriend.

Parents of homosexual or bisexual teens often immediately blame themselves and wonder what they did wrong. They can be hostile to the adolescent, or react with grief, as they begin to realize that many of their own dreams (for the child's marriage, grandchildren, etc.) will not occur.

Happily, there are some differences in the experiences between the adolescents of the early 1970s and before and teenagers coming of age now, in the 1990s. Although antihomosexual feelings are still rampant in North American society, more information and connections are available in society. More recently, homosexual and bisexual teens have the opportunity to safely find each other by contacting the National Gay Task Force.

There is no doubt that the societal stigma of being bisexual or homosexual is an enormous burden for teenagers. In adolescents, and also in adults, it involves ongoing choices about whether or not to be open about your sexual orientation, as new situations arise. While the consequence of passing for straight can be feelings of emotional distance from others, the financial and social costs of coming out and facing discrimination are real as well. These are important choices which must be made.

However, the homosexual or bisexual child who has learned that touch equals love, who trusts others, who has empathy, high self-esteem, and good social skills, who had permission to explore, and whose family handled power well clearly arrives at adolescence with much better tools to experience sexual pleasure, to integrate sexual pleasure with love and intimacy, *and* to face the societal challenges ahead.

> *I still felt close to my parents during adolescence. The house was tiny, it seemed, and there were lots of times where I wished I could somehow get more space, physically. I remember times of frustration, when I didn't want to be bugged, or asked questions. But I loved them.*
>
> *They were so warm and open-minded about life that lots of my friends enjoyed hanging out at my house and just talking to them—especially to my mom. She had a way of really being interested in me and my friends, in what we were thinking and feeling. It was like she was excited by all of the changes going on in our minds.*
>
> *I hadn't figured out I was bisexual yet, and I wasn't really being genitally sexual with anyone. When I finally figured out my sexual orientation, in my twenties, my parents were upset at first, but they came around eventually. I think the fact that I felt close to them for so long helped me to weather the period where I upset and distressed them. I have to say, it was horrible.*
>
> —Roger, 49

Your First Time

Some studies show that the "typical" American adolescent in the 1990s has intercourse by the time he or she is fifteen years old, while other research indicates that only 68 percent of girls and 78 percent of boys had had intercourse by age nineteen.

There is no such thing as a "perfect" first time, but some situations are more ideal than others.

> *And at this point, I knew what he wanted, and I just didn't have the energy to say no, and so we just did it in the car. It was okay. He came right away. It certainly wasn't the way I wanted to have my first sexual experience, but it wasn't traumatic.*
>
> —Jenny, 53

My first time, I was thirteen, and there was a neighbor across the way who used to arm-wrestle with me. She was a little bit older than me. And so we were fooling around in my parents' basement, and we did it there.

—Greg, 41

Well, I was in my second year in college, and I swear, I was the only virgin I knew. And I had been going out with Walt for several months, and I thought he was really sexy. And I just got tired of being a virgin, and I just decided to kind of turn the whole virgin badge in. And so I did. And it was good.

—Gillian, 24

I felt pressured by the rest of the guys. I just wasn't into trying to lay every girl around. I was really kind of shy. But I got tired of the pressure, and I finally went out with a girl who had the reputation of being a tramp. I tried to do it with her, and I couldn't, and I felt really humiliated. I was afraid to try again for years. It wasn't until I was in college and really fell in love with the woman I eventually married that I had good experiences with petting. And so the first person I slept with was also the last—my wife.

—Jay, 38

Clearly, having your first experience with intercourse or partnered genital sexuality with a person who cares about you and will listen to your wishes is an important ingredient in a good first time. Early experiences with intercourse as an adolescent can be very important in forming your feelings about yourself as a sexual person, good or bad.

Natalie and Jim's first time was close to an ideal experience. At seventeen, they had been going out for six months. They had met each other in high school band several years before, and had always liked each other. They had similar interests, including sports, music, and acting. Both came from families that were loving. Natalie's parents had been relatively open about discussing sexuality. Jim's were somewhat avoidant about sexuality but generally supportive.

Nat and Jim had been getting closer and closer physically, with necking and petting, and they felt they loved each other. They were even discussing college choices, in the hopes that they could stay together.

They began talking about whether or not to have intercourse several days before they actually did it. Separately, one spring day,

Natalie went out to the drugstore and bought a foam contraceptive. Jim went a few days later and bought condoms, without knowing what Natalie had done.

On their next date, they discovered what they had each bought. They drove to a "lover's lane," parked, and made love. It wasn't a perfect experience—they were both a bit unsure of what they were doing—and they laughed a lot about it, afterward. They continued to see each other for the next year and continued to have intercourse, with more and more pleasure.

Unfortunately, they wound up going to separate colleges. But both of them felt good about themselves, about each other, and about sexuality because of this first experience. Each of them went on to other successful sexual relationships.

Sexual Trauma

Sexual experiences in adolescence, especially forced or unwanted ones, are very influential in determining adult sexual identity and functioning. Unfortunately, during this time of life, coercive sexual events are very common, particularly for girls.

> *Every time I think about the sexual stuff I did with Todd when I was fifteen, I feel sick to my stomach. Just sick. I was a total dope. He really used me. He manipulated me. And the thing that really bothers me is that I get these sexual flashbacks now during sex with my husband, whom I love, and it really ruins it.*
>
> —Gila, 58

There are various types of unhappy sexual experiences you may have had in adolescence, ranging from being irresponsible and promiscuous to being sexually abused to being coerced or raped. Negative sexual experiences in adolescence happen to both young people who have had basically healthy sexual development thus far, and to those who have already experienced sexual problems and roadblocks.

Sexual exploitation and assault does not happen only to teenagers who are in abusive or neglectful families. It occurs to boys *and* girls—gays, straight, or bisexual (Lobel 1986). Even if your parents were basically caring, sexual trauma can occur, though there are certain ingredients in family life which encourage skills that can prevent adolescents from becoming either the exploitive or the exploited one in sexual relationships:

- feeling valued for oneself, and understanding one's worth as a person

- learning to talk about your desires, rather than simply acting them out

- learning the difference between assertive and aggressive behavior

- growing up in an environment where one's feelings are respected

- discouraging passivity and submissiveness in girls

- growing up with parents who treat each other well

- not being exposed to gender role stereotypes which feed into date rape myths (for example, not hearing women called "cheap")

- having frank discussions about the increasing sexual urges felt by adolescents and how to handle them (including teaching both boys and girls that their sexual excitement is their responsibility, talking about masturbation as a safe way to handle feelings of sexual excitement, and realistically discussing with girls the fact that boys will try to pressure them for sex and teaching them to be assertive in refusing activities which they don't want)

- learning that it is not a good idea to "get high" on a date, since 75 percent of date rapes involves drugs and alcohol

- learning that sexual impulses are healthy and fine, but that partnered sexual behavior should occur only when it is mutually wanted in a relationship (including teaching boys that at *any* point in a sexual interaction, "no" means "no")

- knowing that you are still emotionally connected to your parents and that they will help and support you in any situation, even if you have engaged in forbidden or foolish activities

Many of us were not blessed with a parent who could protect us—a parent who was lucky, vigilant, connected emotionally, open enough about sexual matters, and not afraid of asserting control and influence.

Patsy came from a close family with a very attentive mother. Sexuality was easily discussed in her family, but being sexual at a young age clearly wasn't taken lightly. In ninth grade she went to a new high school, and met a crowd of kids who were much wilder than the intellectual ones she normally went around with. There she met a new guy, named Val who was very interesting, offbeat, and smart. He drank, but to Patsy, that was very exotic. He was handsome, and he kissed really well. He also was a romantic, who recited poetry and went out of his way to walk her home at least once a week, a long distance.

One day, when he walked her home, he met Pat's mother. She noticed that he had liquor on his breath. She also noticed the lusty way he looked at Patsy. Patsy's mother forbade her from going out with Val. This was something that her mother had never done before, and it angered Pat. Naturally, she disobeyed, and one day she went to Val's house after school. Val began to drink, and he got very sexual—more sexual than Patsy felt was right. All of a sudden, her mom's voice rang in her ears, she sensed the danger, and Pat tore herself away, and walked the long walk home.

Sexual trauma, such as date rape or stranger rape, can happen to anyone. Unfortunately, if your family didn't handle your sexual development well, the chances of having traumatic sexual experiences in adolescence, such as rape, seduction by an older person, promiscuous sex, or participating in sexually exploitative relationships increase

Families that don't give children a sense of love, trust, and empathy produce adolescents who are prone to addictions and fleeing from home before they have the job and social skills to take care of themselves. A child who grows up feeling unloved by her parents may grow into a teenager who trades sex for love. A girl who is not allowed to assert her own wishes in an authoritarian home won't have the practice in refusing to do what her boyfriend wants. A boy who doesn't have practice talking and negotiating can't talk his way out of the social pressure to "get laid" by a prostitute, even though he thinks the idea is repulsive. Families environments which were seductive encourage adolescents to get into sexual activities prematurely. A teenager who hasn't been allowed to develop good social skills and have deep friendships is more likely to miss the cues that he or she is being used by another person sexually.

The aftereffects of a traumatic sexual experience in adolescence can be depression, lowered self-esteem, fear, self-hatred, a lifelong distaste for sex, and the whole range of sexual dysfunctions—including lack of arousal, sexual pain, difficulty with orgasm, avoiding certain sexual activities which are associated with the traumatic experience, or subconscious feelings that anyone who likes sex is bad or evil.

Just as Lou, fourteen, was beginning to be interested in girls, and they in him, he was seduced by his alcoholic stepmother (aged thirty-two). She performed oral sex on him, which felt good while it was happening, but afterward, he felt ashamed and dirty, and fled the house. He wound up becoming a male prostitute to survive. For a few years, he lived with an older homosexual man who supported him. It took him fifteen years to pull himself together, get a good job, and be independent.

He met Julie when he was thirty-two, fell in love and married her. Their sex was okay before they got married—but once they got married, he became more and more turned off by her. Whenever Julie wanted genital contact as well as affection, Lou was filled with disgust, and thought of her as a whore. Because his guilty and upset feelings about being used sexually as an adolescent have never been resolved, Lou now feels all sex is dirty.

While too much sexual repression, fear, and guilt is detrimental to sexual development, so is its opposite: too much sexual freedom. In alcoholic, drug-dependent, or neglectful families, parents lack the discipline and energy themselves to set and enforce intelligent rules for their childrens' social adventures. The lack of parental guidance and limit-setting is often viewed by the teenager as a lack of interest.

Sharon began psychotherapy to deal with her depression. Sharon had escaped from a rather disordered past and felt like a phony, living a normal life when in fact she had been a "tramp." She avoided sex with her husband, much as she loved him.

Sharon was a middle child of seven children. Sharon's dad was an alcoholic. Sharon's mother, who meant well and was affectionate, was overwhelmed. She basically let the kids run wild. The siblings were close, and even though the house was chaotic, they felt able to bring their friends around. Sharon was a friendly, outgoing kid by nature, and was comfortable with other children. She was bright and funny, and she liked hanging around with her older brothers and sisters.

Sharon really couldn't count on her mother to take care of the business of living throughout childhood. The siblings depended mostly on each other.

When Sharon was fourteen, she was allowed to go off with a group of eighteen- and nineteen-year-olds, for an entire summer, to a beachfront community one hour away from home. Of course, she had sex all that summer, sex to which she consented. And it spoiled her identity. She feels "cheap" and cannot get rid of the feeling that she is an impostor, even though she is now a successful professional in her own right. While she loves her husband, she is not interested in the sexual part of their relationship.

Ideally, sexual contact and sexual intercourse occur in the context of the natural, gradual unfolding of your own sexual impulses. But a common, emotionally confusing sexual scenario particularly for females is getting into a relatively long-term sexual and emotional relationship with an older person. In this scenario, the older person pushes along the sexual contact and it becomes an accepted, standard part of the relationship (see Alana's excerpt below).

This may have happened to you, particularly when there was a lack of emotional closeness at home, and you used sexuality as a way of getting into a relationship which would get you away from your parents.

If this happened to you, you probably won't think of yourself as having been raped. But the danger is that you will grow up to think of yourself as a person without your own sexual longings and of sexuality as something you do for other people.

Alana (see also page 82) came into sex therapy with her husband, Rich. They have been married for five years and although Alana loves Rich, she doesn't want to have sex with him. She has never experienced sexual desire.

Alana's mother was mostly critical, often controlling, and never talked to her about sexuality. Her father was somewhat distant and was not happy with Alana's performance at school.

Alana wasn't that popular. She hadn't had many experiences with boys. Nor had she had much of a taste of any kind of sexual experience, including exploration of her own body. Once she remembers kissing a boy and feeling her body get "twitchy," but that was the extent of her sexual consciousness.

At fifteen, Alana was just chafing at the bit. She wanted out from underneath her parents' thumb. She wasn't sure what her plans would be for the future; school didn't seem to hold much promise. It was at this time she met Troy, six years her senior.

For the first time in her life, Alana felt like "somebody." She could ride around in Troy's car, after school, and get out of her house. She was so happy to finally have a sense of herself.

Troy began pressuring her for sex soon after they met. He took Alana to a clinic in a run-down section of town to get birth control. She remembers the clinic with disgust—it smelled funny, and she felt dirty and cheap going there.

She has no memories of the first time they made love, and some of her memories of the rest of their sexual experiences together were uncomfortable for her. She didn't feel sexual enjoyment or desire. Troy wanted her to give him oral sex, and sometimes he would hold her head down by his penis and force her. She had intercourse because Troy wanted her to, because she felt it was inevitable, because she didn't want to lose him (and be a nobody again). She went along with whatever sexual activities he proposed, without paying attention to her own feelings of what was okay and what wasn't. Whatever occurred, and she doesn't have that many memories, sex was frequent over the two years they were together.

Talking in therapy, in retrospect, Alana still can't imagine, as a teenager, openly talking to anyone about how to handle her disturbing, ashamed feelings about their sexual relationship. According to Alana, her mother would just have criticized her. And at that time, she didn't want to leave Troy.

As an adult, Alana turned into an assertive, competent woman. It is painful for her to look back on this relationship: "I was trapped . . . passive. And I'm not generally like that . . . I feel naïve, and used. I was so stupid." She blames herself for being passive. She really shouldn't keep criticizing her adolescent self, because what happened wasn't solely her responsibility.

Alana is extremely inhibited in the different sexual practices she'll consider: "I can't help it. I just feel like some of that stuff is dirty, disgusting. It has nothing to do with love." She can't imagine having sexual urges herself. "I know that other women are like that, but not me. I'll never feel that way."

Given the current culture, which objectifies women and glorifies male sexual conquest, how likely is it that a twenty-one-year-old boy would *not* pressure an attractive fifteen-year-old for sex? In Alana's case, her parents saw that she was dating a much older boy, and that he had a car, but they said *nothing* to her about her sexuality and relationships. The omission was so obvious, it must have felt to Alana like her parents were glad to get rid of her.

Even though all of us felt grown up at the time, looking back, it should be clear that as adolescents we were not prepared to protect ourselves from sexual assault or exploitation. In the United States, even currently, there is little sex or "rape prevention" education available publicly.

It takes an open relationship, superb communication, and active intervention, and some good luck, to help a teenage child extricate herself from a situation in which she might be sexually exploited.

And what about boys like Alana's boyfriend Troy, who treated girls like he did? Some of you male readers might look back now, and feel terrible about some of the girls you exploited. If Troy's parents had been open enough to talk about sex in the context of relationship, to talk about sexual urges, and to talk about masturbation, perhaps Troy would have been less likely to be so exploitative.

Male Sexual Myths

Sexual socialization in the United States, just as in many other countries, contains a double standard perpetuated by numerous sexual myths. According to Zilbergeld (1992), some of the most prevalent male sexual myths are that men should never express vulnerability, that sex equals intercourse, and that a man always wants and is always ready to have sex.

Traditional gender socialization for boys gives permission for sexual curiosity and experimentation, as long as it is strongly heterosexual in its definition (Masters et al. 1975). Conventional socialization for boys permits, and even encourages, the expression of sexual drive outside of any relationship context. In *Masculinity Reconstructed* (1995, 13), Dr. Ron Levant lists seven traditional male norms. One of them is "sex disconnected from intimacy."

Bolton, Morris, and MacEachron (1989, 16) go further, commenting, "It is difficult to overestimate the impact of same-sex peers on . . . sexual socialization. . . .[they define] masculinity as sexual aggressiveness through initiation and perpetration."

Psychologist and author Dr. Gary Brooks (1995) illustrates these themes in his article "Rituals and Celebrations in Men's Lives" (1995, 6):

"When I was eleven, my family moved from a tiny town in Maine to a large, multi-ethnic, working class suburb of Boston. As a native, 'hick' kid, I was bewildered by the fast-paced life I encountered . . . I soon learned that the mechanism for proving myself was the ritual street-fight. This wasn't a bloody or dangerous thing, but more of a brief wrestling match. Lots of posturing, but very little real action (thank God!). This wasn't exactly the welcome wagon, but at least it provided human contact and a sense of place in the pecking order.

Years later, having established myself in this group, I was witness to anouther curious transition ritual—'getting laid.' In this neighborhood, many of the older guys enjoyed pressuring the younger ones to venture into the 'combat zone' of Boston, seeking out one or more prostitutes. Many of the guys entered the world of interpersonal sexuality in a half-drunk state, massed together in a cold tenement room, taking turns to get a few minutes of dispassionate sexual thrusting. Most reported more fear and distaste than arousal and sexual gratification. Passion and sexuality were out of the question."

Again, here is the socialized myth that men always want sex. In fact, researcher Dr. Charlene Muehlenhard (1989) has found evidence that young men engage in sexual intercourse when women make advances even when the boys don't want to. This phenomenon occurs because the boys felt they needed to gain more experience; they were worried about their reputations and felt peer pressure; they needed something to talk about; or because they didn't want to appear shy, fearful, homosexual, or impotent.

And despite the fact that females are more likely to be the victims of sexual assault (outside of prison), males can be victims of trauma as well (Bolton et al. 1989; Hunter 1990). Male socialization discourages sensitivity and the admission of weakness (Levant 1995), leading to male victims of sexual abuse and trauma to be less likely to ask for help (Finkelhor and Baron 1986).

Female Sexual Myths

Traditionally, girls are taught to be compliant, to do what they are told, to be friendly and helpful, and to be pleasing to men. They are not taught to be concerned with sexual pleasure, but with "romance"—the notion that they will attract, fall in love, be swept off their feet, and be taken care of by a man. While girls are taught about reproduction, they are discouraged from learning about the parts of their bodies, or about the sexual pleasure they can give themselves (Heiman and LoPiccolo 1988; Kitzinger 1983).Thus many heterosexual adolescent girls are left totally unknowledgeable about their own bodies and erotic feelings, and led to believe that their sexuality will be awakened, lovingly, by a boy.

Ironically, this traditional socialization is a script for disaster. Research (Muehlenhard and Linton 1987) has shown that girls are much more likely to be exploited sexually by boys if they are taught to be sweet, passive, compliant, and to think of sexuality as "something your husband will teach you." (Dr. Muehlenhard has concluded that girls should steer away from men who have sexist attitudes, men who insist on making all the decisions about what will happen on a date, and men who refuse to take "no" for an answer.)

But for most women, their parents did not constructively confront these twin realities: the positives of their sexual coming of age and the negatives of traditional male sexual socialization. There was no acknowledgment that it would be good to get to know their own bodies, sexually. And when girls were warned about men, it was done in a very frightening, sex-negative way.

Ideally, parents would have modeled respect, love, and affection, in their relationship, and would support their daughters developing a loving relationship with a boy. At the same time, they would be realists and would have prepared their girls for the kinds of lines they would be fed by heterosexual boys who were merely looking for a sexual conquest. (For instance, Sol and Judith Gordon's *How to Raise Conservative Kids in a Sexually Permissive World* (1983) gives advice for how to prepare daughters to fight lines such as: "If you loved me, you would", "What's the matter, are you frigid?", "You have to. You got me this excited", and "I paid for everything; you owe it to me.")

The clash of male and female socialization left many adolescents vulnerable to sexual experiences which created sexual scars-in many cases, this misinformed myth-perpetuation provided the societal backdrop for date and acquaintance rape.

Date and Acquaintance Rape

Most rape, and specifically most acquaintance rape, happens between the ages of fifteen and twenty-five. During dating, young people are faced with the pressures of sexual encounters, usually without any experience or guidance in knowing how to deal with them.

With teenage and young adult males biologically driven and wanting sexual relationships, adolescent and young adult women can easily get caught up in dating relationships in which there is sexual coercion, and become victims of date or acquaintance rape.

Studies (Ageton 1983; Levy 1991; Koss et al. 1987; Abbey et al. 1996) have shown that between 20 and 25 percent of college women will experience rape or attempted rape at some point in their college careers. In addition, the uncensored contemporary opinions of a shocking percentage of bright, well-educated young men are compatible with beliefs that underlie sexual assault, exploitation, and rape (Koss 1988; Goodchilds and Zellman 1984; Muehlenhard and Linton 1987; Koss and Harvey 1991). Study after study has shown that quite a few boys think that forced sex is permissible in certain situations, such as when the girl initiated the date, when the boy paid for the date, or when the couple went back to the man's home or car. Much research indicates that if a girl has done anything which the boy feels has "led him on," he has the right to sex. So, once a girl agrees to have sex, if she later changes her mind and doesn't want it, some boys feel that it is acceptable to force the intercourse. In addition, some justify coercion if they are so turned on that they don't believe they can stop.

In almost every rape situation, even in situations where the victim was drugged, there is misplaced self-blame.

> Karen came from a very traditional, modest, sex-avoidant Italian family. Her father was the head of the house. Sex was not discussed at all, nor was any aspect of relationships with boys. She was shy and had had very little experience dating. She was bright, and friendly, but quite naïve.
>
> She went off to college and wound up in a coed dorm—with coed bathrooms! In addition, unbeknownst to her, the dorm in which she was placed was known as a "party" dorm. There was a lot of drinking going on, not just on weekends but during the week, too.
>
> One night, one of Karen's male dorm-mates invited her into his room to talk. She knew him from several classes, and she didn't think anything of it. While there, she had a few drinks. She believes that this boy put some kind of sedative into her drink because she became very woozy. The next thing she knew, she saw two other boys in the room. They forced her to perform oral sex on all three of them.
>
> Karen is happily married now, but she still has intrusive memories of her sexual assault. She feels guilty, as if she did something wrong, even though rationally, she realizes that these young men were simply rapists.

> Dara went to high-school in an upscale neighborhood outside of New York City. Her family was very successful financially but wasn't terribly empathic or close.

Dara didn't feel understood or valued in her family. Her mother was self-absorbed and critical and seemed competitive with her. Her father was prone to fly into rages in which he verbally abused everyone in the family, including the mother and the kids. Sexuality wasn't discussed much in her family, but there was a lot of concern about looking successful and having many friends.

Dara had lots and lots of friends. One evening, after going to a football game, she and her group began drinking quite a bit. There was one boy who was there that evening with whom she had flirted recently. She didn't know him well. The group decided that they would split up for a while, and then meet up at one of Dara's girlfriend's houses later.

She went off in a car alone with this new boy. They wound up driving around and then making out and petting heavily in a parking lot until late at night.

It was really too late to meet up with her girlfriend, and this boy was pressuring her for more sexual activity. Dara said no. He threatened to drop her off, alone, in the lot where they were parking. But it was the dead of night and it was cold. She was scared, and couldn't think straight.

Dara was afraid to walk all the way back, alone, to her friend's house, where she was supposed to sleep over. And she felt it was so late that she would get her friend in trouble with her parents if Dara showed up in the wee hours.

Dara did not feel that she could go to her own house, which was about three miles away. She smelled of liquor. It was late. She just knew her father would scream at her. She couldn't take it.

So she got back in the car with this kid, and he took her to his house. His parents were asleep already. He had his own suite in the lower part of the house. As she walked down the stairs to his room, he barked at her to take her clothes off and get on her hands and knees. She felt really humiliated; she had never ever gotten into that physical position with a boy. She protested, refusing to take most of her clothes off, and he persisted.

She was scared but she took off her clothes. She told him that she didn't want to have sex. She began to cry. He entered her anyway, and began slamming himself into her from behind. She kept crying. He was saying, "My cock is really big, huh!" She kept crying and he kept on raping her. Afterward, he acted astounded that she was still weeping. At that point, he finally realized what he had done, and he began to cry, too.

Dara never even told her mother about this incident, because, as she puts it, when she tells her mother something distressful, her mother just yells at her for upsetting her. At thirty, Dara still thinks sadly of this incident, and she still blames herself for it.

Recovery

Recovery from sexual assault or from bad feelings left over from exploitative or unwise sexual relationships takes time and courage, but it can be done. There are different degrees of trauma, and some of you should not attempt this task alone.

If you had adolescent incidents which left you with spoiled feelings, but your previous sexual development had gone well, you may be able to do a lot of reparative work on your own.

But if what happened was a major incident (such as rape or sexual abuse), involved violence, if you are still having flashbacks, or if recalling the incident is too painful to stand, you should seek professional help. The same is true if you often feel depressed, fragile, isolated, not grounded (in reality or in your body), or like you cannot cope with life. Do not do this work on your own.

However, under any of these circumstances, you still can learn about the components of the healing process, and you still can begin thinking about what you want to change. Doing the exercises at the end of this chapter will help you figure out what to target in therapy. But though you can write down what happened to you, do not elicit vivid memories about it until you are in treatment with a professional.

Mental health experts have done a lot of research and made great strides in treating sexual trauma just in the last few years (Resick and Schnicke 1992; Westerlund 1992; Shapiro 1989 and 1995; Vaughan et al. 1994; Smythe 1995; Korn 1997). So if you carefully choose a competent psychotherapist with up-to-date training in working with sexual trauma, psychotherapy can help you change your distorted attitudes about yourself and your sexuality. Even if the trauma happened long ago, it is likely that you can be helped to get over it today.

The key to beginning the healing process rests in dismantling the fear and disgust and in incorporating a new, positive outlook about your future sexuality. This involves several stages (Smythe 1995).

1. Stop avoiding the fact that the incident(s) happened.

2. Write down your ideas about why the event occurred the way it did.

3. You need to become clear on your faulty, negative beliefs about sexuality that are based in the adolescent trauma.

4. You need to choose a new, positive set of beliefs about the experience.

Negative sexual events which occurred in adolescence can create great anguish. Many survivors of such events do not attempt to change at all, and just suffer with their changed self-esteem, depression, changed associations to sexuality, sexual avoidance, sexual pain, or sexual dysfunction (Golding 1996; Resick and Schnicke 1993). It isn't necessary to live your life with sexual pain, without ever experiencing sexual pleasure, or with abridged sexual pleasure, because of what happened to you in adolescence.

If you suffered from unwise, exploitative, or traumatic events in your adolescence, the exercises at the end of this chapter will help you begin to reclaim your sexual self.

If You Need Professional Help

If you fit the description of someone who needs professional help (see Recovery section, page 194), use what you have written in your journal so far to consciously change what you say to yourself when you think of these troubling sexual incidents. Find a competent professional to help finish your trauma work.

Becoming an Adult

It is much better to grow up in a family where both parents accept an adolescent's changing identity, budding beauty or handsomeness, and emerging sexuality. When your parents give you feedback that your awakening sexuality is normal and not dangerous, and that they still love you in your new incarnation, it helps you to cement a healthy sexuality.

One of the tasks of adolescence is to consolidate this newfound sexuality into your new identity as an independent person. Being a sexual person does not necessarity mean having intercourse, and it certainly doesn't mean being promiscuous. It *should* mean feeling permission to be alive, experiencing your sexual stirrings at your own pace, learning to feel good about your sexual self, and mastering how to give yourself sexual pleasure without hurting yourself or others.

Whatever problems you had in your life prior to adolescence, don't get stuck blaming yourself for calamities you had in your teenage years. There are societal and familial forces answerable for the widespread existence of adolescent sexual trauma. By learning to make a *reasonable* assessment of what happened (dividing up the responsibility and putting it in context), forgiving yourself, and working on developing good feelings about being a sexual human being, you will begin on the road to a healthy sexual life.

Exercises

Examine Your Adolescence

List three *nonsexual* critical incidents, or family themes, positive or negative, which stand out in your mind as defining your unfolding adolescent sexuality. You can refer to your journal writings for other chapters to review early issues of family development such as touch, empathy, trust, power, friendship, and family environments. Also think about the major themes of adolescence, like your changing body, your relationship with your peer group, your parents' reaction to your sexuality, and your socialization. (If you experienced sexual trauma in adolescence, write those incidents in the "Reassign Responsibility for Sexual Trauma" exercise on page 197.

1. _____

2. _____

3. _____

What are the consequences of these incidents today, in terms of your belief system, sense of your sexual self, or feelings about sexuality as an adult?

Theme or Incident   **How It Affected My Adult Sexuality**

_____

_____

_____

List the changes you would like to make in these areas. Think in terms of correcting beliefs or behaviors.

The Incident or Theme   **The Current Behavior or**
                                             Belief I Will Change

If You Were Sexually Active As An Adolescent

If you were sexually active as an adolescent and/or experienced sexual trauma, complete the following exercises you believe pertain to you.

Reassign Responsibility for Sexual Trauma

If you experienced sexual trauma in adolescence, complete the steps below. If you experienced more than one incident, make a copy of this sheet and complete one for each separate incident.

Describe the incident here:

How did you originally feel about the incident?

_____

_____

What familial factors, if any, do you believe contributed to the incident(s) occurring (for example, low self-esteem kept me from leaving; my bad body image made me too afraid no one else would have me; etc.)?

_____

_____

_____

_____

Which sexual socialization factors do you believe may have come into play?

_____

_____

_____

_____

Looking at all the factors you have named, write a new assessment of responsibility for the episode: Divide up the responsibility for the factors, some to the person who hurt you, some to your family background, and some to yourself.

_____

_____

_____

_____

Regrettable but Consensual Relationships

If you were in a consensual sexual relationship as an adolescent, and you regret your actions, answer the following questions. If you had more than one, make a copy of this sheet and complete one for each relationship.

What did you get out of this relationship at the time?

In retrospect, what do you wish your parents had said to you, or asked you, about this relationship?

Do you think them addressing the problem would have helped you to stand up for yourself or fix the relationship, or do you think you would have stayed in it anyway? Why?

Choosing What You Would Like to Change

Once you have reexamined your adolescence, and sexual and nonsexual events that have caused you to view sex in a negative context, you need to choose what you wish to change.

List any bad feelings you have about sexuality in general, and also about *specific* sexual acts, that you might have because of your adolescent experiences.

Bad feelings I have about being sexual in general:

_____

_____

_____

Bad feelings about participating in specific sexual behaviors which are linked to bad adolescent sexual experiences:

**Things I now feel are dirty
or disgusting**

**The events which I
associate with the acts.**

_____

_____

_____

You are in control of your sexuality now. Mark with a "C" (for "change") any activity you now shun which you would like to feel fine about.

Identify Negative Beliefs

Frequently, after a traumatic event, your whole inner model of life changes in a very negative way, and then you go on to organize your future life around that negative belief system. Read the following list of some common negative beliefs (Shapiro 1989, 1995; Westerlund 1992; Resick and Schnicke 1993; Korn, 1997) and check off any that apply to you. If you have a negative belief which isn't listed here, write it down.

Negative beliefs:

_____ I am never safe.

_____ I am in danger.

_____ I must be in control of myself and relationships at all time.

_____ No one can be trusted.

_____ I can never let myself relax sexually again.

_____ I can never trust anyone/men/women again.

_____ I am worthless.

_____ Sex is dangerous, sick, disgusting.

_____ I am not good.

_____ I am powerless.

_____ I will always be a sexual victim.

_____ I deserved the bad consequences which happened when _____

_____.

_____ Physical intimacy is impossible for me.

_____ _____ (write in a particular behavior) is disgusting.

Write any other negative beliefs here:

_____

_____

_____

Mark with a "C" (for "change") all of the beliefs you would like to change.

Replace the Negative with Positive

Thinking of how your sexual life has been constrained by what happened to you in adolescence, check off the positive beliefs you would now like to incorporate into your world view and your sexual self.

Positive beliefs:

_____ I can learn to trust others.

_____ I can take care of myself now.

_____ I deserve good things.

_____ I did the best I could.

_____ I was young and inexperienced. I can forgive myself.

_____ I was young and inexperienced then. I can take care of myself now.

_____ It's over. I'm safe now.

_____ I'm okay. It wasn't my fault.

_____ I can learn to make good choices in people.

_____ I can protect myself now.

_____ I can emerge stronger.

_____ It is normal for me to have sexual needs and desires.

_____ I can begin to explore my body.

_____ I can allow myself to feel sexual feelings.

_____ My taste in foods has changed over the years. I can learn to enjoy different sexual activities, too.

_____ Sex is becoming easier for me.

_____ My sexual sensations can flow freely.

_____ Sexual feelings can please me.

_____ I'm beginning to like my sexuality.

Write any other beliefs here:

_____

_____

_____

With a colored pen, write a "G" (for "goal") next to the beliefs that you would like to adopt first. (Pick the easiest ones to start with.)

Now write down here your plan for integrating some of these positive beliefs (i.e., your corrective beliefs, a soothing mantra, or your plan to read a book).

_____

_____

_____

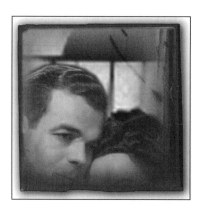

Chapter 11

The Effect of Physical Violence on Sexuality

Most Americans cling to the image of the family that includes tranquillity, happiness, love between members bound together by blood and/or legal ties, certainty of behavior, shared norms and values, and above all, safety . . . despite the fact that the media has increasingly shown the "underside" of family life . . . More violent crimes occur in the home than outside its doors; and more violence occurs between family members than among strangers.

—Mildred Pagelow, *Family Violence*

◆ **Did you witness physical violence between your two parents?**

◆ **Did a parent harm you with physical violence?**

◆ **If such violence occurred, are you bothered by any of the following symptoms?**

- chronic anxiety

- changed associations to touch

- an inability to relax and be in your body

- an inability to "lose control" in any situation, because the world feels "unsafe"

- depression

- an inability to trust others

- **an inability to enjoy being sexual**

- **a fear of an intense sexual and emotional bond to a lover or mate**

- **sexual dysfunctions or lack of desire**

The United States is a violent country. While family violence is commonplace in North American society, it remains a somewhat hidden problem. Having had a history of nonsexual physical violence in one's family is a common, unrecognized cause of adult sexual problems.

The statistics are shocking. A 1988 report by the American Bar Association estimates that 3.3 million to 10 million children witness domestic violence each year, and that in nine out of ten cases, the victim is their mother. Noted sociologists Straus, Gelles, and Steinmetz (1980) determined that there was physical abuse of children in three out of five homes. Because of different ways of defining child abuse, other estimates of physical child abuse vary widely, ranging from 60,000 to 1.5 million children abused each year.

But what might be the correlation between having experienced physical violence as a child and adolescent and sexual problems in adulthood? This chapter looks at the relationship between growing up with family violence and sexual inhibition. If you grew up in a family where your parents hit you, or hit each other, or your siblings were violent, you have a whole host of negative associations to relationships, control, marriage, touch, trust, love, and sexuality. Many of these associations are unconscious, creating sexual barriers that may be difficult to overcome. But, once you make the link between your past exposure to violence and your sexual problems, with patience and commitment, there are steps you can take to feel more comfortable being sexual and intimate.

Conceptually, the results of different kinds of family violence—being a victim yourself or being a witness—are different, but the ways in which they negatively affect sexuality are quite similar.

I do think my problems trusting women, being intimate, and being sexual are related to what happened in my family. My father constantly beat my mother, and he beat us, too. My mom was so overwhelmed by him and what he did to her that she couldn't protect us.

He was a maniac, just uncontrollable. I can remember walking home, and just dreading going to the house. I knew he'd find some reason to thrash me. He'd beat me with a belt until I bled, or knock my head into the wall. And she did nothing to stop it. It was like she was frozen.

At times, I know that my anger at her for not protecting me makes me suspicious of all women. And then other times, I get all confused, because I felt as a kid, and I still feel now, that I should have been able to save her. So I feel guilty.

One incident I'll never forget. He was drunk as usual and I could hear him beating her. Over and over again. And then, it was winter outside, it was snowing, and he tore her clothes off of her, and he pushed her outside on the porch, naked. And he yelled at her, "This is where you'd be, if not for me." I overheard and saw the whole thing. I was seven. I felt I should have been able to stop him, but I was so afraid of him that I couldn't get out of bed. And so I just lay in bed, listening to her cry.

—Glen, 28

Acting Out or Acting In

Growing up with physical violence tends to be so disturbing to one's sense of emotional safety and bodily integrity that most victims of violence avoid directly confronting its reality. Although there are no hard and fast rules about how a child might react, scientists studying the effects of family violence on children have found a tendency for boys to "act out"—reacting by doing things in the outside world, e.g., being aggressive, and for girls to "act in"—to internalize their feelings (Wolf 1988; Wolfe and Starr 1988; Starr and Wolfe 1991).

Some adults who experienced family violence "act out" sexually. For them, growing up in an unempathic and violent home environment leads to sexual addiction (see chapter 9), and/or a sexual style of using people, without ever becoming emotionally attached to them. Although women can and do "act out" sexually, the pattern seems more common with men.

In worst case scenarios, the combination of parental lack of empathy and family violence creates adults who are so terrified of equal relationships with others that it can lead to the development of aggressive sexuality and paraphiliacs—for instance, voyeurs, exhibitionists, frotteurs, and obscene phone callers, as well as criminals who violently attack others sexually (see chapter 9).

Suffering family violence may lead to "acting in," which can take the form of depression or the inhibition of sexuality as an adult. Both men and women can react by "acting in," and having difficulty with sexual desire, arousal, or pain disorders.

Joani grew up in a family of six kids. Her alcoholic mother had no patience to take care of the children's needs, and she lost her temper and hit and pinched them on a daily basis. As the youngest child, Joani sometimes was protected by her older brothers and sisters, but it was a frightening environment. Joani's father was a banker, and he left home for work every day. All of the kids tried to get the father to admit to the mother's pattern of physical abuse, but the father kept up his denial. He focused his attention on making money, because his main goal was that his children "succeed and go to college." By the time she was in high school, Joani was alone with her mother's wrath. She couldn't stand it, and left home without finishing high school.

Joani eventually got her G.E.D., went to community college, and went on to become a dental hygienist. She fell in love with one of the dentists she worked for, and they got married. But Joani had no sexual desire whatsoever, and her husband insisted that they go into sex therapy. The connection between her lack of sexual desire and the history of family violence became clear to her when she looked at her BodyMap (see page 29) and realized that she had no areas of green on her body. She realized that she was afraid of touch and linked love, fear, and abandonment.

Ryan was fifty and had never been married. As a child, he had been beaten and kicked by both parents, and the violence continued until he left home at eighteen. He didn't trust anyone, and put all of his energy into making a success of himself financially. He became a skilled insurance salesman, but continued to reject offers of friendship and companionship from women. He didn't feel comfortable initiating either physical or sexual relationships and had no sexual desire. He finally sought psychotherapy for his loneliness. When he made the link between the violence in his family and his inability to trust others or feel good in his body, he slowly began to be able to reach out to women.

Depression

Although the sexual consequences of growing up in a violent home usually are not discussed, the other negative results are. According to researchers at the University of Michigan, growing up in a violent home as a child is particularly likely to lead to bouts of major depression in adulthood. In a survey of 2,867 adults, Ronald C. Kessler, Ph.D., at the school's Institute for Social Research, along with colleague William Magee found that people with a family history of violence are about two and a half times more likely to get depressed by the time they are twenty than those who haven't experienced the violence. After age twenty they're twice as likely to get depressed—and have twice as many bouts of depression.

Repression, Denial, or Playing Down

If you were a victim of violence and have managed to cope and make it into adulthood without academic or work problems, obvious psychiatric problems, or overt addictions, your survival into "normal" adult life probably depended on using repression, denial, or playing down of the prior physical abuse or violence (e.g., "That's just how kids were raised in those days"; or "All of the husbands and wives in the neighborhood where I grew up had these kinds of violent fights. It's not so unusual"). You grew up believing that what you experienced was normal. But no one from a violent home truly escapes unscathed. Usually, functioning in at least one important area of living, like the ability to work, to love, or to enjoy sexuality, is impaired.

> *Well, I don't really consider what my mother did as abuse. We lived in a big apartment building and during the summer, when all the windows were open, you could hear what was going on in all of the families. Lots of other kids were being slapped around, too. My mother wasn't anywhere near the worst. That's just the way people thought you should discipline. It was the 1940s.*
>
> —Brad, 62

Research (Starr and Wolfe 1991; Jaffe, Wolfe, and Wilson 1992) shows that children from violent homes often suffer with seemingly unrelated problems, such as headaches, abdominal pains, stuttering, bed-wetting, and sleep disturbances, or depression, anxiety, suicidal tendencies, phobias, withdrawal, academic problems, poor relationships with peers, or lowered self-esteem. As an adult, you may have anxiety, depression, or long-standing sexual problems.

Identifying Oneself as a Victim of Violence

Frequently, clients come into sex therapy wanting help but not making the connection between the nonsexual family violence they met with growing up and their sexual problems. Lately, the media has publicized the obvious connection between childhood sexual abuse and later sexual dysfunction, but the interrelationship between nonsexual violence and adult sexuality is not generally discussed in books, magazines, or on TV. Clients who were physically but not sexually abused, and clients from families where a parent was physically abused frequently "forget" to share this information with their therapist. The therapist may not catch the omission by not asking about violence (unless she routinely uses a violence checklist such as the Ratner checklist in appendix B.)

What might make a client accidentally "forget" to reveal witnessing or experiencing physical abuse? Psychologist Angela Browne (1991) discusses how challenging it is to consciously confront the fact that growing up in your family did you great harm.

> Defining oneself as the victim of a family member may . . . require significant and painful alterations in the victim's perceptions of the perpetrator and of themselves. Victims talk about the devastation of trying to incorporate the realities of assault and blatant disregard for their well-being into their images of parents or adult partners who profess to love them, or who are at least in the roles of those expected to love, nurture, and protect. . . . Further, our society frequently is intolerant of those who bear the label of victim. Victims are seen as weak, unable to handle daily life effectively, out of control, and nuisances. They are often viewed as responsible, at least in part, for their victim status; or are avoided because their pain and anxiety and the responsibility for involvement with them makes others uncomfortable.

I never really consciously thought of myself as a victim. After all, I'm over six feet tall, and after I got to junior high, my dad wouldn't really dare to beat me. But now that you mention it, I guess that some of the irresponsible behavior of my teen-age years, the drinking, the drugs, and those two times I totaled the car and almost got killed, I guess that was what I used to avoid focusing on what was going on in the family around me.

—Kyle, 51

Conflicting Emotions

Being the victim or the observer of family violence is confusing—often the abused child may still feel loyalty and love toward the parent. Even the worst parent is, at times, loving and kind. Dr. Mildred Pagelow (1984, 25) has commented, "The pattern of intermittent reinforcement of tender caring and closeness before and after beatings is probably one of the important factors that keeps victims emotionally bound to their abusers."

> *She was neglectful and abusive most of the time. I still have a scar on my elbow, from when she threw me into a wall when I talked back to her. And you know, on rainy days, that damn thing hurts like the dickens. . . .*
>
> *Well, it wasn't as if it was all bad, though. She loved me, in her own way. She tried, sometimes, to do nice things for me. I remember once, she saved up what was a lot of money at the time to buy me a special jacket I wanted. And another time, she complimented me on a cake I baked her, especially for her birthday. I think I even have a picture of me taken with her, proudly showing off that cake. It makes me sad to think that that was the last time I really felt she loved me, and I think I was about nine years old.*
>
> —Freda, 58

Because the gender role behavior for men dictates being strong, men have an especially hard time looking at what occurred to them as victimization.

Bud began sex therapy complaining of lack of desire and some erectile problems. He couldn't understand why his sex drive was so much less than his peers. He had no interest in quickie sexual relationships with girls he didn't care about. While girls were very interested in him and flirted with him, being cavalier about sex didn't feel right. At the same time, his lack of interest in recreational sex set him apart from his peers and made him feel like he "wasn't quite a man." This thought only made him more fearful, and whenever he wanted to make love, he was filled with anxiety about whether or not his penis would stay erect.

Only when he began examining the details of his parents' relationship did he begin to understand his deep conflicts about male/female relationships. Bud was involved with a woman he liked very much, but he wasn't sure that he would be able to make a long-term commitment to her.

As a small boy, he saw his father act violently and controlling toward his mother. At one point, he recalls seeing his father smash his mother into a wall. Another time, he saw him drag her around by her hair. Bud tried unsuccessfully to get in between them several times to protect his mother. In reviving these memories, he felt a surge of sadness and helplessness. Once he uncovered the link between his parents' violent relationship, his protectiveness toward his mother, his defenselessness toward his father, and his fear of hurting his girlfriend (and therefore being, in his mind, an awful man like his father) his sexual problems diminished.

Sexual Development: The Fallout

Almost all of the developmental tasks described in *Sex Smart* may be difficult to master if you grew up in a home with physical violence. Perhaps most damaging are the changes in associations to touch. As mentioned in chapter 1, at the base of satisfying adult sexual pleasure is comfort with touch and sensuality. Soothing touch is an avenue to relaxation. The unconscious link between soothing touch and safety allows human beings to loosen body boundaries, an ingredient in powerful sexual bonding. Yet in a family in which people hit each other, and maybe even threaten to kill each other, touch has a different message: danger, pain, betrayal, and fear.

Betsy recalled the memory of being five years old and touching her father's arm to calm him down when he flew into a fury. Even as she did it, she was disgusted by touching him and aware that she wasn't doing it out of love, only out of trying to subdue him.

James suffers chronic anxiety. He was beaten frequently by his father, and doesn't feel any pleasure in his body at all. He feels jumpy all the time. When his girlfriend touches him, it doesn't feel good, it just tickles. He can't relax enough to enjoy sensual pleasure. His girlfriend is often angry at him, because when he has sex, he just likes to get erect and enter her. He doesn't feel comfortable with hugging or kissing.

James's father used to hit him on the head, neck, and shoulders. Touches in those areas upset him, and when Julie, his girlfriend, tries to throw her arms around him, his first impulse is to hit her. Although he doesn't strike her, sometimes he freezes up physically, and he can't respond warmly.

As a child, Suzanne was beaten, beaten, pinched, and kicked so severely that she is now "tactily defensive." Suzanne's sense of touch has been ruined. Almost no sensation on her skin is pleasant. She can only wear certain kinds of fabric, and loose clothing styles that skim her body. She is so hypersensitive to touch that she has a hard time being physically close with her children under the best of circumstances. On hot, suffocatingly humid days, when it is hard to breathe and her childrens' skin is sweaty on hers, she cannot stand to touch them at all. She has no interest in having sex with her husband.

Post-traumatic Stress Disorder

Living with chronic family violence is a major, life-threatening traumatic event from which some victims never recover. One psychiatric disorder which frequently develops as a result of chronic family violence is post-traumatic stress disorder (PTSD).

According to the American Psychiatric Association (1994, 209–11), post-traumatic stress disorder might occur if a person was exposed to a traumatic event under two conditions: "(1) the person experienced, witnessed, or was confronted with . . . events that involved actual or threatened death or serious injury [to] self . . . or others," and; "(2) the person's response [was] intense fear, helplessness . . . horror [or (in a child)] disorganized or agitated behavior."

If the above is true, PTSD is the diagnosis if certain criteria are met. First, "[t]he traumatic event is persistently reexperienced in one (or more) of the following ways:

1. recurrent and intrusive distressing recollections of the event, including images, thoughts, or perceptions. . . .

2. recurrent distressing dreams of the event. . . .

3. acting or feeling as if the traumatic event were recurring (includ[ing] a sense of reliving the experience, illusions, flashback episodes, including those that occur on awakening or when intoxicated). . . .

4. intense psychological distress at exposure to internal or external cues that symbolize or resemble an aspect of the traumatic event

5. physiological reactivity on exposure to internal or external cues that symbolize or resemble an aspect of the traumatic event"

Second, the person evidences "[p]ersistent avoidance of stimuli associated with the trauma and numbing of general responsiveness (not present before the trauma), as indicated by three (or more) of the following:

1. efforts to avoid thoughts, feelings, or conversations associated with the trauma

2. efforts to avoid activities, places, or people that arouse recollections of the trauma

3. inability to recall an important aspect of the trauma

4. markedly diminished interest or participation in significant activities

5. feelings of estrangement from others

6. restricted range of affect (e.g., unable to have loving feelings)

7. sense of a foreshortened future (e.g., does not expect to have a career, marriage, children, or a normal life span)"

Third, the person shows "[p]ersistent symptoms of increased arousal (not present before the trauma), as indicated by two (or more) of the following:

1. difficulty falling or staying asleep

2. irritability or outbursts of anger

3. difficulty concentrating

4. hypervigilance

5. exaggerated startle response

In addition, by definition, the "[d]uration of the 'symptoms' is more than 1 month" and "[t]he disturbance causes clinically significant distress or impairment in social, occupational, or other important areas of functioning."

Hypervigilance and Exaggerated Startle Response

If you are a survivor of childhood family violence, you may evidence indicators of PTSD such as scanning, bodily anxiety, a need to stay in control, hypervigilance, and an exaggerated startle response. "Hypervigilance" is when you never let your emotional or physical guard down—you are always scanning the world, watching for danger, and you feel you must stay in control at all times. An "exaggerated startle response" is when you jump when any noise or a touch surprises you. These symptoms may interfere with or sometimes entirely block sexual desire or sexual pleasure.

Gerd came into therapy complaining that he had trouble with low sexual desire and maintaining erections.

Gerd can't lie down and go to sleep easily, and he can't stretch out and relax: he taps his fingers or moves his legs nervously. He has a lot of trouble enjoying sexual relations, if his wife wants to initiate, because he can't unwind and enjoy touching.

Gerd had an easier time when he was younger, and his biological sex drive was higher. He had a lot of spontaneous erections back then. But now that he is older, with a body that isn't so driven for sex, he needs to be able to relax and focus on pleasurable sensations in order to get an erection, and he has difficulty letting go and trusting and relaxing.

When he thinks about his difficulties with sexuality and relaxation, his memories go back to childhood. His father beat his mother frequently, and sometimes he beat Gerd, too. If Gerd's father was out drinking, sleep was impossible. If he was home, maybe Gerd could sleep. As a kid, Gerd remembers not going to sleep right away, but instead, pacing up and down, until he fell asleep from exhaustion.

Gerd recalls that his mother "never slept." She was in a "watchful state all night." Even now, years and years after the divorce, Gerd's mother still can't get a good night's sleep.

Gerd's early experiences with a chaotic and dangerous family environment created difficulties with being able to relax and feel safe, physically, within his environment and within his own body. Now that he is older, and his constant physical urge to be sexual has lessened, these problems are coming to the fore.

Take a look at the self-soothing and relaxation section of chapter 2. Re-read the floating exercise on page 40, where you are asked if you can imagine relaxing on land or floating in a protected setting on the water. If you are hypervigilant, this is a frightening image.

Researchers working on PTSD have found that even a single traumatic event can change the brain's chemistry. During trauma, the body automatically shifts to a "fight or flight" response: The heart rate races, the pupils dilate, and blood is sent racing to the muscles. In PTSD, the shift to "fight or flight" can be induced by anything that even faintly resembles the original trauma. In fact, sufferers may not be aware of what has triggered their reactions (van der Kolk 1986).

> John, who had been severely isolated, beaten, bullied, and terrorized by his father throughout his childhood and young adulthood, wrote on an assessment questionnaire that he had had a "happy" childhood. He had never married. He never expected anything good to happen to him in life, and tended to notice all evidence of betrayal and danger in the world around him. Even though his father was quite feeble and in a nursing home, John was plagued with the feeling that somehow, his father's evil energy was all around him, and that somehow, his father would still be able to harm him.

In one study, reported in the January/February 1992 issue of *Psychology Today*, researchers found that trauma victims secrete an important stress hormone called CRF. Because of the presence of too much CRF, they react to emergencies that do not exist in the present moment. Therefore, extreme fear reactions triggered by seemingly minor causes may be the result of the original trauma that was experienced.

Based on these research findings, if you grew up with family violence, you may have some of these PTSD symptoms without even being conscious of them. Obviously, this has major consequences for your experience of sexuality. Even though your physical state may be one of chronic anxiety, you don't know it! This is the only body you have ever had, and this is the only way you have ever lived. You may not necessarily sense that your chronic levels of tension, "jumpiness," and inability to relax are negatively impacting your life (especially your sex life) and are alterable conditions.

> In therapy, as James finally began to admit how terrifying his childhood was, he realized that he still feels anxious when he hears arguing, particularly if he can't actually hear what is being said. He also feels scared when he hears clinking ice cubes—the sound reminds him of how his father imbibed drink after drink and powered himself up to start a physical fight.

Susan began sex therapy complaining of vaginal pain and low sexual desire. There was evidence of emotional neglect and physical violence between her alcoholic mother and her father, and on her BodyMap, Susan's whole body was blue and red, except for some green on her neck. In fact, she liked her husband to put his arms around her neck and hug her.

When discussing the lack of bodily safety evidenced in her BodyMap, Susan recalled memories of being at her parents' house when her parents were fighting: glasses whizzed past her ear, knives were pulled out and brandished, broken glass was everywhere. Even though she was just a little girl, she was the one who tried to stop her parents, often stepping right into the fray. She remembered repeatedly locking herself in a bedroom with her smaller sister, protecting her sister with her own body. She remembers telling her sister, "Don't worry, it will stop soon." Susan shielded her sister from the violence and the danger, but no one shielded Susan.

Once Susan was able to acknowledge and not minimize the true trauma, chaos, and danger of her past life, she began to practice relaxation techniques and creating a SafePlace (see chapter 2). As she looked realistically at the security of her current life with her loving husband, her ability to relax and feel pleasure in her body increased, and her vaginal pain abated.

As noted in chapter 2, trust that the world is predictable and that the people in it will meet your needs is crucial for sexual unfolding. Unfortunately, unless you concretely address your chronic sense that the world is dangerous, and rework the past trauma, your anxiety is likely to increase. Since life is full of ups and downs, if you are inclined to focus on the negative, life's experiences will just leave you feeling more distrustful and cynical. Use the exercises at the end of this chapter, as well as the exercises at the end of chapter 2, to work on your anxious body.

The feeling of being totally safeguarded comes from a secure childhood with a consistent, available caretaker. To some degree this is an illusion (in fact, good parents are not omnipotent, they cannot keep a child from contracting a dreaded disease, or from getting hit by a car), but it is a helpful illusion. If touch reminds you of the safety of the mother-child bond, than it is a shortcut to relaxation and solace (see chapter 2). If your family life has been marked by emotional and physical betrayal, your whole sense of safety may be marred.

Sandra, whose mother had been physically abusive, had difficulty with arousal and orgasm. She had done months and months of work in psychotherapy on letting go of her body "armoring"—the chronic physical tenseness she carried in her. As her tension abated, she allowed herself to enjoy being sexual.

One night, she went to very deep levels of arousal and connection with her husband, Dave. The first time this happened, she was frightened that she had let down her guard with Dave so dramatically without consciously telling herself that that was what she wanted to do. Later that week, she dreamed a terrifying vision that her mother was chasing her. She ran to safety by going to a "safe place" that she had worked hard to establish at the beginning of her therapy.

Sandra subconsciously felt that if she let down her vigilance in any area, even being orgasmic with a loved partner, she would become overly trusting, too vulnerable, and would be hurt again.

Role Reversal: Children Acting as Parents

Children of battered spouses are likely to have experienced role reversal. (Since 95 percent of battered spouses are women, "mother" will be used here.) If you felt you had to step in and defend your mother, then you lost the feeling that your mother could protect you. You developed what some experts in violence call "pseudomaturity"—you acted like the mature adult in the situation, even though you were a frightened child (Jaffe et al. 1990).

Research has shown that battered women suffer from many kinds of physical and emotional disorders (for example, depression and anxiety). At times, your mother acted confused and disoriented, unable to act like a protective parent, as a result of her persistent fear (Walker 1984). And because the average woman earns much less than the average man, even if your mother tried to protect herself and you by leaving her abuser, your situation in life might not have improved much. Researchers have found that a child of a battered woman is more likely to have been exposed to other life stresses, such as multiple separations from friends and other loved ones, poverty, poor housing, overcrowding in shelters, and frequent home and school moves. As a child-witness, your pseudomaturity in the face of real danger probably caused body armoring. This kind of childhood role-reversal can lead to a problem with trust and letting go in intimate relationships.

Betsy had witnessed brutal wife abuse, and had taken care of her battered mother through most of her childhood, contributing to difficulties in sexuality as an adult. She began therapy with complaints of anorgasmia. She was tense, felt numb, and complained that all touching tickled her. Her BodyMap had very little green. Betsy grew up with an extremely violent and abusive alcoholic father. When he drank, he would threaten to kill her mother. He pulled guns on Betsy's mother with regularity. He beat Betsy's older sister. Enraged, he once drove his car through the wall of her house into their living room.

Betsy's mother was caught up in the cycle of abuse, where after a beating, her husband was tender and acted repentant. She couldn't get the strength to leave the relationship. She felt unable to make a living and her husband was a good provider.

Because she felt her mother was more fragile than she herself was, Betsy never complained or acted scared—she tried to be in charge. Betsy was her father's favorite, and since he never hurt her, she felt responsibile for calming her father down, to keep him from hurting either her mother or her sister.

When Betsy began to acknowledge the true trauma of her violent past, a lot of rage and resentment emerged. However, she was surprised to find that as she began to express her vulnerability verbally, her need to be physically armored diminished. Her "ticklishness" subsided, she found more areas in which she welcomed touch, and her sexual pleasure increased.

Growing up in a violent family has a huge impact one's gender identity. As mentioned in chapter 4, in developing our own sense of gender identity, we rely on our parents as models. When children are abused by parents, their associations to the gender of their abuser are harmed, as are associations to the gender of the parent who stood by and let the beatings occur. In witnessing spousal violence, children are essentially forced to pick between an identification with the abuser or with the victim! Denial of the reality of the horror of family life is probably more common among adults from violent families than is conscious integration of the truth. And with denial comes repetition.

Research has shown that boys who grow up with violent male models are more likely to become batterers themselves in adulthood than are boys from non-violent families (Pagelow 1984). Yet many male children of male batterers do reject their fathers' model of masculine behavior.

But even if you were conscious of how disastrous the violence was during childhood and adolescence, your ideas about gender still were negatively impacted. Betsy, grew up to feel that all women are weak. Betsy's sexual imagery was damaged as well—she recalled that even in the midst of the most abusive periods in her life, her mother would continue to have sex with her father. Betsy was determined to be a different kind of woman than her mother: to act strong, to not become sexually attached, and to not let herself become dependent on a man.

Bud, who we also met in this chapter (pages 210–11), associated masculinity with violence. Bud felt that he had to be completely sensitive to the women in his life at all times to not be a male monster like his father. For Betsy as well as Bud, problems identifying positively with their own gender caused sexual difficulties.

The role of adequate self-esteem in developing healthy sexuality was discussed in chapter 5. If your parents frequently fought violently, neither of them was paying consistent attention to their children's needs for empathy, socialization, or supervision. In an atmosphere of chaos, the environment is "every man for himself," and sibling relationships may also have been marked by conflict. Additionally, your self-esteem was affected by the shame you felt in living in a dysfunctional family.

If you were abused yourself, by one or both parents, then you may have viewed that as evidence that you are worthless. The pain of not having been protected by the very people who are supposed to love you the most was overwhelming (Browne 1991).

In chapter 6, themes of power and control and how they become woven into the ways each of us expresses ourselves sexually were discussed. Families where parents are authoritarian and not empathic can produce children who link love and control in a way that prevents sexual intimacy as adults. As described in chapter 9, child victims of violence and abuse may subconsciously link sexuality and fantasies of revenge. They are too fearful of other people to be able to tolerate egalitarian relationships. In the worst case scenario, they may develop a pattern of masturbating and having orgasms to sadistic fantasies, and then go on to "acting out," thus becoming sexual criminals.

If you were a victim of family violence, your sexuality may have beeen changed to an overriding focus on power, but it is more likely that you have dealt with this threat by "acting in" instead of "acting out". Having experienced physical violence often leads to sexual inhibitions and dysfunctions. One common theme is that sexual attraction is dangerous, because it can lead to powerlessness. A second phenomenon is a sense of not wanting to share one's body.

Deanna came into couples therapy with her husband, Eric. They loved each other, but often got into terrible power struggles and verbally vicious, circular fights. Also, Eric really liked sex, and Deanna wasn't interested.

Deanna came from a family where the parents physically slammed each other, and her mother often hit her. She got used to living in a state of chronic anxiety; it became "normal."

Her parents fought so much, and so physically, that she often walked home from school and wondered if she would find them both alive that evening, or whether one of them would have killed the other. As an adult, she was left with generalized anxiety, and was always on the lookout for something going wrong.

Through her childhood and adolescence, it seemed that no matter what the stimulus, the response was always some form of hitting. She came home one day from a serious bike accident, with a five-inch gash in her leg, bleeding profusely. When Deanna dragged herself up to her apartment for some tender loving care, her mother took one look at the blood all over her, the wound, and her blood-stained clothes and smacked her across the face.

Deanna left home early to marry, looking forward to some peace and to being her own boss. However, her assertive and somewhat dominant husband pushed all of her old buttons, and she was determined that she would not let him control her. She could not allow herself to enjoy being sexual with him. To begin with, it was difficult to relax. But in addition, she felt that sex equaled subjugation, and she was certainly not going to be one-down in a relationship again. It took many months of sex and marital therapy, integrating how violence affected her development, for Deanna to realize how much she loved her husband and for her to be open to the sexual part of their relationship.

Hayley came from a cold, distant family with a strict pecking order: the father ruled the mother, the mother ruled the kids. The mother hit and slapped the children, in order to get them to do what she wanted. There was always work to do, and the girls in the family had to help with all of the cooking, cleaning, and washing.

Money was tight. There weren't enough possessions to go around. Hayley, as one of the younger kids, only got to wear hand-me-downs. One day, Hayley won a book at school for being such a good student. She proudly walked home and showed the beautiful, new book to her mother. Her mother promptly took the book away from her, saying that they already had a copy of it, and that in the future, one of the kids could use it as a gift when invited to a party. Hayley cried, and her mother responded with another slap.

When she grew up and got married, Hayley never felt comfortable with touch. In addition, she had strong feelings about not wanting to have sex with her husband. She felt that one of the few things she owned herself was her body, and she didn't want to give it away.

Another major theme for you, if you came from a family where there was violence, is a sense of isolation, and gaps in your people skills. Learning to socialize with others is a crucial step in a child's sexual development (refer to chapter 8). However, violent parents literally believe that they own their children, and they may have kept you from having friendships and connections with others around you. Researchers have found that children of violence have poorer social skills in general (Wolfe et al. 1988; Westra and Martin 1981).

Families where physical child abuse occurs tend to be quite detached from others. Researchers have found that the parents are inclined to move from one geographical location to another, probably to escape from legal troubles. The activities occurring in the house are kept secret. Even if you had friends, you probably didn't want them coming to your house, because you were afraid that your friends might see the abuse that was taking place routinely.

Sandy spent her childhood so cut off from her peers by the violence that she felt awkward socially. Sandy and her mother and brother ran away from their violent father several times—each time going "underground" to a shelter, where they were hidden for many months, which continually interrupted her relationships. She couldn't go to school, and she couldn't tell people where she had been. She felt shame about her father's violence, and she couldn't open up to her friends and tell them what had become of her. She finished high school without any really close friends, and she feels that the experience of social shame, stigma, and isolation has stuck with her in adulthood—she still finds it difficult to make friends.

Assessing the Damage

If you grew up witnessing or experiencing physical violence in your family, your sexuality may have been affected negatively in each of the important developmental stages explored in *Sex Smart*. Most likely, your sexual inhibition has been triggered by this violence.

The exercises at the end of this chapter and the ones in chapter 2 will help you investigate further the violence / sexuality connection and guide you in expanding your ability to take pleasure in emotional relationships, letting go of chronic tenseness, and enjoying unrestrained sexuality.

If your pattern has been to act out sexually, you might want to reread and revisit the exercises in chapters 6 and 9, and look at the resources in the back of the book pertaining to those chapters.

Exercises

Before you start these exercises, make sure you have established a SafePlace and have mastered the exercises in chapter 2. Reclaiming your body is a major task which needs to be accomplished for your recovery sexually, but you need to be able to soothe yourself and create a feeling of safety before you are ready to open up any new imagery about your violent past.

The Violence-Symptom Checklist

Which of these symptoms / behaviors do you think you have? Check off the ones which apply, and give examples from your relationships.

_____   Afraid of assertiveness: _____

_____

_____   Worried about anger in relationships: _____

_____

_____   Concern with boundaries: _____

_____

_____ A fear of dependence: _____

_____ A fear of abandonment: _____

_____ Distrust of others: _____

_____ Concerns with power and powerlessness in relationships: _____

_____ Concern that you must be in control at all times: _____

_____ You feel unlovable, have poor self esteem: _____

_____ Feelings of social isolation or problems with socialization/friends:

_____ Body armoring: _____

_____ Difficulty in relaxing in your body: _____

_____ "Relaxing" creates anxiety, the feeling that you are out of control:

_____ Heightened startle response: _____

_____

_____ Very little sense of pleasure at being touched: _____

_____

_____ Don't want to share your body with anyone else: _____

_____

_____ A high level of general anxiety: _____

_____

_____ Association of love and violence: _____

_____

_____ Distorted gender identification: _____

_____

Assess Your Violent Family History

Using Your BodyMap

Follow the instructions for making a BodyMap on page 29, then do the following:

For all the areas that are colored red, see if you can discover the reasons for your bad feelings of touch. Do you have any violent memories associated with that body part or area? If so, write them down here.

_____

_____

_____

After several months of doing the exercises in chapter 2, redraw your Body-Map. Compare the two maps.

Using Imagery to Confront the Violence

Pick the most violent incident you can remember from your childhood and write down all of the details—anything you can remember: sights, smells, sounds. Replay it. Go back to exercise 1 the Violence-Symptom Checklist, (page 222) and see if you can make any more connections between the violence and your sexuality.

Violence Genogram

Violence often runs through several generations of your family. If you know your family history, draw your family tree, and trace which of your ancestors was violent or abusive to their children.

Changing Your Belief Systems

There are lots of beliefs you may have developed which are creating sexual barriers. Please check the ones which are true, and write a disputing sentence under it:

_____ Violence is normal in families.

_____ The world is dangerous.

_____ I can't believe a woman would actually want to be sexual with a man.

_____ To be a good man, not like my father, I must be sensitive and gentle all the time.

_____ It's not safe to be as dependent on a partner as my mother was on my father.

_____ Women are violent and crazy.

_____ It's not safe to get close to a man

Conquering Bad Dreams

If you are struggling with bad dreams, where your abuser is still torturing you even now that you are an adult:

1. Start keeping a record of any bad dreams you have in your journal. For the first two weeks, just collect data on your dreams.

2. Then, in the third week begin doing this exercise three times a week or more (at least once a day) close to bedtime:

   • Close your eyes and breathe deeply.

   • Imagine the dreaded person shrunk down to the size of a thumb.

   • Then imagine the pitiful menace, shaking their tiny fists and screaming in a teeny voice, looking so pathetic that the situation is humorous.

3. After eight weeks have passed, review the bad dreams you've recorded in your journal and see how they have changed.

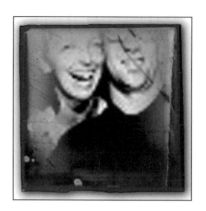

Conclusion

Take responsibility for your own sexual pleasure. As much as you might like to think that someone else will turn you on and give you joyful paroxysms of sexual pleasure, in actuality we are each responsible for our own eroticism. . . . [the] notion of sex as something one person does to the other—or the somewhat kinder notion that sex is something one person does for the other—both can lead to problems. By taking responsibility for your own sensual and sexual needs, you actually are paying your partner a terrific compliment: in effect, you're saying to them, I care enough about you to want to keep you from having to guess at what I want, what I like, and what can make me happy.

—William Masters, Virginia Johnson, and Robert Kolodny, *Sex and Human Loving*

Now that you have completed reading *Sex Smart* and have done the exercises at the end of each chapter at least once, you have begun your journey. You have probably changed some, already, from what you have read and explored.

You have summarized your new understanding of what happened to you at each stage of sexual development in the journal you created. Hopefully, you're beginning to see how the way your family handled issues such as touch, empathy, power, and socialization—not specifically sexual issues—has changed who you are sexually today from who you might have become if things had been different. And you may also see how your parents' handling of the more obvious sexual issues in family life—permission to explore sexuality and masturbation—have affected you for good or for ill. And, you may have a much more in-depth sense of your goals for sexual actualization.

Take some time at this point to review appendices C and D; look again at the medical and relationship factors which might be coming into play in your sexual difficulties. This book only addresses family issues in sexual development. Remember that you must take responsibility for checking out possible medical causes of any sexual problems. If you have not already discussed your sexual difficulties with your physician, you must do so.

From your work in *Sex Smart*, some of you might have only a few areas on which you must work. Others of you may have a lengthy list of goals. If you have a number of objectives, don't get overwhelmed. Instead, think of the work you need to do in stages, and begin working on one developmental issue at a time.

In reading *Sex Smart*, you may have realized some distressing or surprising connections between your family, your past, and your sexual functioning. If what you have discovered is upsetting, you might want to get some support to explore it further. Suggestions for how and when to seek professional help are on page 230.

Look again at the "Milestones in Sexual Development" model in appendix A. At this point, each of the names of the stages has new meaning to you. From your journal entries, you probably can see that certain stages were more central to your own sexual unfolding than others. While the ideas of the book are still fresh, go back and reread those key chapters and look at the resources for each of those chapters. Make a note in your journal about any books, tapes, or courses you would like to pursue. The exercises at the end of this chapter will help you assess what has changed already, and what your new goals may be. If you plan to read this book several times, you might want to make copies of these exercises and redo them each time you reread *Sex Smart*.

> *. . . I feel that I'm getting more open sexually, and now I'm understanding how my family contributed to my developing vaginismus, and my inability to tell Bruce, for all those months, that he was hurting me.*
>
> *Here is the list of things I have come up with in my childhood that I did not have at home: fun, humor, joy, trust, connection with others, unconditional love, commitment, acceptance, support, warmth, feeling of normalcy, sense of permanence about things, carefree feelings, dependence on others, understanding of how things worked between people, communication, honesty, physical or emotional comforting, being wanted, feeling important, special or valuable; responsiveness, consistency, safety. That's a lot longer than I thought it was going to be when I started out.*
>
> —Beth, 35

Seeking Professional Help

As a young adult, a therapist I was seeing gave me permission to be sexual by acknowledging I had sexual feelings I could act on responsibly and appropriately within a loving relationship. I began to enjoy and appreciate sex without guilt with my boyfriend.

—Johanna, 37

Many of you may feel quite capable of proceeding on your own, using the suggestions and resources which have been provided in this book. But if you have profound, unyielding sexual blocks from the early years—in trust, in empathy, or in touch—and you need a lot of encouragement to reach out in the world, you will make progress the fastest if you get professional help. This may also be true if your sexual problems are a result of trauma. Finally, if for any other reason you find that you feel overwhelmed, depressed, or frightened about what you have discovered after reading *Sex Smart*, you should get professional help. In all these cases, your next goal is to find yourself a good sex therapist.

If you are an adult and are still a virgin and want to be less afraid of getting into a sexual relationship, be sure to note the resources on page 253. You will have to decide for yourself whether or not you want to speak with a professional psychotherapist. You may have come from a family which was very loving but very restrictive about sexuality. It may be easier to discover your own attitudes and values about sexuality and implement a plan of change with some outside, professional support.

If you decide to seek expert advice, the exercises at the end of each chapter in this book should give you a sense of the kind of work you need to do in individual psychotherapy. You will need a therapist whose style is active, not one who sits and listens and says very little. You want to find a professional who is willing to guide you through the exercises, one who will intervene and make suggestions, and who will address any resistance you have to doing the work.

You need to like the person, intuitively, and to feel that they like you. It isn't sufficient for them to come highly recommended; you need to feel a connection with them. You need to feel that they understand you.

Ideally, it would be best to begin your work with a professional who is a certified sex therapist. Talking about sexuality is difficult for most people. The general training of most psychotherapists does not prepare them to be sexual therapists.

Within the United States, the credentialing organization with the most stringent criteria is called the American Association of Sex Educators, Counselors, and Therapists, or AASECT. You can contact them at:

P.O. Box 238
Mount Vernon, IA 52314-0238
319-895-8407

AASECT also knows the names of certified sex therapists in some other countries. If you need to contact AASECT and it has moved, or you live in a different country and need to find a parallel organization which certifies sexual professionals, the reference librarian in your local library can help you.

In most places, there is no legislation or licensing which regulates who can and cannot call themselves a sex therapist. Many insurance companies and managed care companies are not consumer oriented, or have restricted panels of providers, and they may refer you to a professional who is not well trained in sexology. Seeing a therapist who isn't well trained often does more harm than good. As an educated consumer, take the time to research local resources when you need additional help for sexual problems.

If you live somewhere where you absolutely can't find a certified sex therapist, you must take a very active role in finding an appropriate therapist. Call the national AASECT office first to ask for suggestions of sexual professionals in your state who might know a good therapist in your local area. Also talk to some of the urologists and gynecologists in your local area, and ask them to whom they send their patients with sexual problems. Then interview some of the professionals whose names have been given to you.

If you find that you have both individual issues and relationship issues, you will have to get some advice from the professionals you interview as to whether it would be best to begin in individual or couples therapy.

In the short term, targeted therapy can be very helpful for many people. But you may need longer term therapy. For that, you will have to pay out of your own pocket, if not right away, then after a while, since insurers no longer want to pay for long-term therapy. If you don't have money, try to find someone with training in sexual issues who works out of a clinic or a nonprofit family counseling organization, who can see you for a reduced fee.

Any struggle you go through to achieve the changes you seek will be worth the work. As you begin to feel more and more comfortable with your own sexuality, you will naturally feel more pleasure in your body. And you will feel happier in general, as well. You'll feel more like you deserve other kinds of pleasures, and your self-esteem will improve. Body, mind, emotions, and spirit are all connected. Alter any aspect of yourself, and every other part is affected. Any change you can imagine clearly, verbalize, or write down is beginning to happen just in the process of making your wishes conscious. Best of luck!

Exercises

Assess Your Goals for Sexual Actualization

Date: _____

Revisit Your BodyMap

Make another BodyMap, following the instructions on page 29, and color it in, thinking of it in relation to being in an affectionate, safe, and relaxed situation with someone you like romantically. Now, compare this Body Map to the first one you did when you originally read chapter 1. What changes are there? Write them here.

_____

_____

What are the areas of touch you want to continue to work on?

_____

_____

Areas to Focus On

Now that you have read the whole book, which areas do you believe have been the most influential in creating sexual barriers for you? Review the following list and place a checkmark by the top three.

_____ Love

_____ Touching

_____ Empathy

____ Trust

____ My Ability to Relax and Be Soothed

____ Body image

____ Gender identity

____ Sexual orientation

____ Self-Esteem

____ Power and control

____ Permission to explore

____ Socialization

Adolescent issues:

____ Masturbation/Sexual fantasy

____ Separation from parents

____ Sexual trauma in adolescence

____ Family violence

Now review the list on page 10. Looking at all the Gs you marked down, pick the four most important goals and write them down here.

1. _____

2. _____

3. _____

4. _____

If you see relationships between the goals you chose and the areas of sexual development, write the connections down here.

My goal	**Relates to (from list on pages 232-233)**

1. _____

2. _____

3. _____

4. _____

Your Action Plan

Write today's date, and write down your action plan for reinventing your sexuality.

_____

_____

_____

_____

Appendices

A

Milestones in Sexual Development

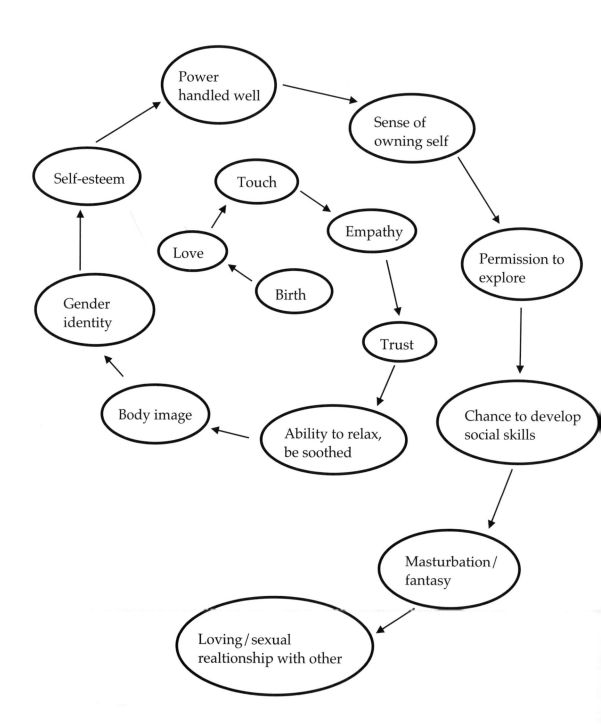

B

Abuse Checklist*

	Happened to me	Happened to others in family
Emotional Abuse		
• Calling you names, constantly embarrassing you/others or putting you down	☐	☐
• Belittling or rejecting you, blocking your attempts at self-acceptance	☐	☐
• Harassing you or making you the object of malicious or sadistic jokes	☐	☐
• Making you steal or do other illegal things	☐	☐
• Blackmail	☐	☐
• Punishing you unfairly	☐	☐
• Making you perform cruel or degrading tasks	☐	☐
• Criticizing your independent thoughts and feelings	☐	☐
• Telling you that you have no right to be alive or that you are unworthy	☐	☐
• Telling you that you are always or usually wrong; dictating religious thoughts	☐	☐

* From *The Other Side of the Family* by Ellen Ratner, 1990.

	Happened to me	Happened to others in family
• Making you feel hopeless	☐	☐
• Punishing you in public or in front of other family members	☐	☐
• Always comparing you to others	☐	☐
• Making you eat something you spilled on the floor	☐	☐
• Deliberately raising you as a member of the opposite sex	☐	☐
• Preventing you from going to school	☐	☐
• Terrorizing or bullying you	☐	☐
• Isolating you from others	☐	☐
• Rejecting you by openly preferring your siblings	☐	☐
• _____	☐	☐
• _____	☐	☐
• _____	☐	☐

Neglect

	Happened to me	Happened to others in family
• Leaving you alone for days or weeks in the care of others	☐	☐
• Ignoring you or not responding to your needs	☐	☐
• Not feeding you or providing you needed clothing, or making you feed yourself before you were able	☐	☐
• Not washing your clothes	☐	☐
• Ignoring your physical needs and/or not getting you required medical attention	☐	☐
• Providing little physical nurturing, such as holding you or talking to you	☐	☐
• Leaving you with an irresponsible caretaker	☐	☐

	Happened to me	Happened to others in family
• Not providing proper nutrition or not giving you enough to eat	☐	☐
• Providing an uninhabitable place to live: drafty, unclean, or unsafe	☐	☐
• Your parents were drug or alcohol abusers and neglected you as a result	☐	☐
• Your parents didn't get out of bed to care for you	☐	☐
• Not allowing you to leave your room or your home for long hours, days, or weeks	☐	☐
• _____	☐	☐
• _____	☐	☐
• _____	☐	☐

Physical Abuse

	Happened to me	Happened to others in family
• Shoving	☐	☐
• Throwing	☐	☐
• Slapping, hitting, spanking that caused marks or bruises	☐	☐
• Scratching or biting	☐	☐
• Burning	☐	☐
• Cutting	☐	☐
• Breaking your bones or making you bleed	☐	☐
• Not allowing you to defecate or urinate	☐	☐
• Tying or locking you up or restraining you in other ways	☐	☐
• Using heat or cold (usually water) to cause pain	☐	☐
• Using rubber bands or other materials in your hair to cause pain	☐	☐
• Holding your head under water or otherwise trying to suffocate you	☐	☐

	Happened to me	Happened to others in family
• Making you sit or stand for unreasonable periods of time	☐	☐
• Using hunger as a consistent punishment	☐	☐
• Confining you to a small space for long periods of time	☐	☐
• Forcing you to eat unhealthy or unsanitary food or food designed for animals	☐	☐
• Forcing you into toilet training too early	☐	☐
• Medicating or drugging you when you were not ill	☐	☐
• Locking you out of the house as punishment	☐	☐
• Forcing you into child labor	☐	☐
• Hurting or killing your pets	☐	☐
• Serving your pets to you as food	☐	☐
• _____	☐	☐
• _____	☐	☐
• _____	☐	☐

Sexual

	Happened to me	Happened to others in family
• Lying nude or being provocative	☐	☐
• Showing you pornographic pictures or movies	☐	☐
• Flirting with you or engaging in provocative behavior	☐	☐
• Kissing, holding, or touching you inappropriately	☐	☐
• Raping you	☐	☐
• Touching, biting, or fondling your sexual parts	☐	☐
• Giving you enemas or douches for no medical reason	☐	☐

	Happened to me	Happened to others in family
• Forcing you to observe or participate in adult bathing, undressing, toilet, or sexual activities	☐	☐
• Making you engage in forced or mutual masturbation	☐	☐
• Forcing you to be nude with others	☐	☐
• Making you share your parents' bed when other beds were available	☐	☐
• Making you look at or touch adults' sexual parts	☐	☐
• Allowing you to be sexually molested	☐	☐
• Telling you about their explicit sexual behavior	☐	☐
• _____	☐	☐
• _____	☐	☐
• _____	☐	☐

C

Medical and Psychiatric Issues

While many sexual problems are caused by social values, cultural taboos, and personal and family attitudes, you should never assume that any given sexual problem you have is strictly "in your mind." Please, go to your internist and be honest about what your sexual issue is, and get a medical workup. You could have a sexual problem which stems from physical causes: structural, hormonal, or neurological. The internist may then make you see another specialist such as an endocrinologist or a urologist. Follow through on the medical investigation.

In addition, your physician may send you for a psychiatric screening. Many psychiatric disorders can affect sexual health and adjustment, including, among others, substance abuse disorders (alcoholism and drug abuse), schizophrenia, and anxiety disorders.

Depression is often linked with low sexual desire. It is crucial that you be carefully screened for depression. Do not assume that you know whether or not you are depressed, since many people do not recognize the many symptoms—including guilt, feeling inadequate, lack of interest in other people, and fatigue.

A cursory answer to a few questions asked by a friend or a physician is not an adequate screening. Research has shown that depression (and other psychiatric illnesses as well) are under-diagnosed by primary care physicians (Goldberg 1995; Von Korff et al. 1987). You need to take a valid test, such as the Beck Depression Inventory (Beck 1979).

There is a complex interaction of biology and emotion in sexual chemistry, and ironically some antidepressants as well as some drugs which you may have been given for other medical conditions can inhibit desire, cause erectile problems, block orgasms, or affect sexual functioning in other ways. In some cases, your physician may have failed to warn you of these negative sexual side effects. One good resource for researching whether drug side effects might be causing your sexual problems is *Sexual Pharmacology: Drugs That Affect Sexual Function*, by Crenshaw and Goldberg (1996).

Trained sex therapists know that a medical and psychiatric screening is crucial before proceeding to treat sexual problems on the theory that the problem is based on cultural, family, emotional, or relational factors. When you use this book, you have to take responsibility for getting a medical and psychiatric screening.

D

Relational Factors Checklist

Sex Smart is about familial factors that impact your sexuality. If you're having sexual problems within a relationship, you need to also think about *another* potential source of many sexual problems (such as lack of desire, or erectile problems, or orgasmic difficulties): your relationship.

Your *motivation* for being sexual within an ongoing relationship is your emotions about that other person. If you don't feel good about that other person, there is a strong possibility that you won't feel much like being sexual with them.

Here is a list of *some* of the reasons you or your partner might not be able to function sexually in the relationship:

_____ Problems with general communication, talking, and conversation

_____ Not feeling the person is on your side

_____ Money and financial matters

_____ Problems with different values, activities, or lifestyle issues

_____ Lack of quality time together

_____ Disagreements over issues with each partner's family of origin

_____ Feelings/conflicts about domestic roles and responsibilities

_____ Lack of attention and affection

_____ Unresolved anger from old fights

_____ Power and control issues in general

_____ Domestic violence, tempers, or general hostility

_____ Work problems

_____ Arguments over child rearing

_____ Problems with ex-spouses or stepchildren

_____ Jealousy

_____ Trust

Do you have problems in many of these areas with your partner? On the whole, these days, do you have more bad feelings than good ones about your partner? If so, there is a very good chance that some part of your sexual problem is a relationship problem.

E

Anger Episode Record

Date: _____   Time began: _____ am / pm

                              Time ended: _____ am / pm

	mild		moderate			severe			extreme	
Anger level	1	2	3	4	5	6	7	8	9	10
Aggression	1	2	3	4	5	6	7	8	9	10
Impact	1	2	3	4	5	6	7	8	9	10

Symptoms/signs: *physical tension*   *agitation/irritablity*
                     building sensation   *clenched fists*
                     quickened breathing   *violent/physical image*
                     raised voice

Anger-provoking thought / situation: _____

_____

_____

What I said or did: _____

_____

_____

Anger-reducing thoughts: _____

_____

_____

Alternative behavior: _____

_____

_____

F

Developmental Factors Contributing to Inhibited Sexuality in Persons from Physically Violent Families

Basic Trust	Fear of dependence / Abandonment
	Fear of intimacy
	Possible role reversal with victimized parent / Issues of pseudomaturity
	Poor ability to be comforted
Problems with Touch	Chronic inability to relax / "jumpiness" / Exaggerated startle response
	Changed meaning of touch
	Disturbed body map / Lack of pleasure in the body
	Disturbed bodily sensations: numbing, ticklishness
	No sense of owning own body
Depression	Hopelessness; pessimism
Anxiety	PTSD symptoms
	Chronic anxiety: vigilance, scanning
	Afraid to "lose control"
	Inability to soothe self

Gender Issues	Distorted gender identification Does not want to identify with gender of abuser Does not want to identify with gender of victim
Overconcern with Power and Powerlessness	Concern that sexual connection will lead to power-lessness Worries about boundaries, possessions Frightened of "giving in too much" or of asking for things

Socialization Issues	Social isolation
	  • Parent intentionally kept child from social contact with peers
	  • Child felt ashamed of chaotic, dangerous family; afraid to invite guests to house
	  • Victimized adult flees to shelter or new location, taking child along. Child loses continuity with peers.
	Poor social skills
	Poor conflict resolution skills
	Difficulty in accurately labeling feelings, communicating

Poor Self-esteem	Feel defective, unworthy
Negative Beliefs That Interfere with Intimacy	"Violence is normal in families." (Denial) The world is unsafe, dangerous "I can't believe a woman would actually want to be sexual with a man."

Resources

Chapter 1

Gach, M. 1997. *Acupressure for Lovers*. New York: Bantam.
If you are very uncomfortable touching and being touched, you will have to try many different methods of expanding your comfort skills. It is very important to go at your own pace. Try this book once you are past the "beginners" level with touch.

Independent Video Services
401 East 10th Ave., Suite 160
Eugene, OR 97401-3317
800-678-3455
Wendy Maltz, M.S.W., has produced two outstanding video tapes that are an ideal starting point for helping you to become more comfortable with touch: *Relearning Touch* helps increase basic skills in communicating through touch. It is appropriate for each reader of *Sex Smart* (45 minutes/$89.95 plus $5.00 for shipping and handling). *Partners in Healing* helps couples identify sexual problems caused by childhood incest (43 minutes/$79.95 plus $5.00 shipping and handling).

Acupressure Institute
1533 Shattuck Ave.
Berkeley, CA 94709
800-442-2232; 510-845-1059
If you are comfortable with both touch and seminudity, you may want to order some of Dr. Michael Gach's videotapes available through the Institute.

American Art Therapy Association
1202 Allanson Road
Mundelein, IL 60060
897-949-6064

American Dance Therapy Association
2000 Century Plaza, suite 108
Columbia, MD 21044
410-997-4040

International Expressive Arts Association
P. O. Box 641246
San Francisco, CA 94164-1246
415-522-8959

Chapter 2

Davis, M., E. R. Eshelman, and M. McKay. 1995. *The Relaxation and Stress Reduction Workbook*, 4th ed. Oakland, Calif: New Harbinger Publications.

Douglas, J., and F. Atwell. 1988. *Love, Intimacy, and Sex*. Newbury Park, Calif: Sage.

Hazan, C., and P. Shaver. 1987. Romantic love conceptualized as an attachment process. *Journal of Personality and Social Psychology* 52:511–524

Chapter 3

Freeman, R. 1988. *BodyLove: Learning to Like Our Looks and Ourselves*. New York: Harper and Row.

Heiman, J., and J. Lo Piccolo. 1988. *Becoming Orgasmic: A Sexual and Personal Growth Program for Women*. New York: Fireside.

Hutchinson, M. 1985. *Transforming Body Image: Learning to Love the Body You Have*. California: Freedom Press.

Markway, B., C. Carmin, A. Pollard, and T. Flynn. 1992. *Dying of Embarrassment: Help for Social Anxiety and Social Phobia*. Oakland, Calif.: New Harbinger Publications.

Reinisch, J. 1990. *Kinsey Institute's New Report on Sex*. New York: St. Martin's Press.
This book gives excellent information about what is "normal" and on aspects of body image which can and cannot be changed.

Wolf, N. 1991. *The Beauty Myth*. New York: William Morrow.

Wolf, S. 1993. *Guerilla Dating Tactics*. New York: Dutton.
To push yourself out into the dating scene, no matter what you look like.

Zilbergeld, B. 1992. *The New Male Sexuality*. New York: Bantam.

Chapter 4

Brooks, G. 1995. *The Centerfold Syndrome: How Men Can Stop Objectifying Women and Achieve True Intimacy*. San Francisco: Jossey-Bass.

D'Augelli, A. R., and C. J. Patterson, eds. 1995. *Lesbian, Gay and Bisexual Identities Over the Lifespan: Psychological Perspectives*. New York: Oxford University Press.

Kitzinger, S. 1983. *Women's Experience of Sex*. New York: Penguin.

Levant, R., with G. Kopecky. 1995. *Masculinity Reconstructed: Changing the Rules of Manhood*. New York: Dutton.

Money, J. 1980. *Love and Love Sickness: The Science of Sex, Gender Difference, and Pair Bonding*. Baltimore: Johns Hopkins Press.

Money, J., and A. Ehrhardt. 1972. *Man and Woman, Boy and Girl*. Baltimore: Johns Hopkins Press.

Reinisch, J., and L. Rosenblum, eds. 1987. *Masculinity-Femininity: Basic Perspectives*. New York: Oxford University Press.

Chapter 5

Branden, N. 1987. *How to Raise Your Self-Esteem*. New York: Bantam.

Heiman, J., and J. Lo Piccolo. 1988. *Becoming Orgasmic: A Sexual and Personal Growth Program for Women*. New York: Fireside.

McKay, M., and P. Fanning. 1992. *Self-Esteem*, 2nd ed. Oakland, Calif: New Harbinger Publications.

Zilbergeld, B. 1992. *The New Male Sexuality*. New York: Bantam.

Chapter 6

Davis, M., E. Robbins Eshelman, and M. McKay. 1995. *The Relaxation and Stress Reduction Workbook*, 4th ed. Oakland, Calif: New Harbinger Publications.

McKay, M., P. Rogers, and J. McKay. 1989. *When Anger Hurts: Quieting the Storm Within*. Oakland, Calif.: New Harbinger Publications.

Miller, A. 1983. *For Your Own Good: Hidden Cruelty in Child-rearing and the Roots of Violence*. New York: Farrar, Straus & Giroux.

Potter-Efron, R. 1994. *Angry All the Time: An Emergency Guide to Anger Control*. Oakland, Calif.: New Harbinger Publications.

Also, make a copy of appendix E on page 249 and fill out the Anger Episode Record to start gaining control of your anger now. If you are not successful within a short time, seek behavioral treatment from a professional with experience in working on issues of anger control.

Chapter 7

Give yourself permission to learn about your gender socialization and sexuality by reading books that give you a wide range of information you may have missed during your youth and adolescence.

McCarthy, B. 1988. *Male Sexual Awareness: Increasing Sexual Satisfaction*. New York: Carroll and Graf.

McCarthy, B., and E. McCarthy. 1989. *Female Sexual Awareness: Achieving Sexual Fulfillment*. New York: Carroll and Graf.

For Survivors of Negative, Oversexualized Family Environments and Sexual Trauma:

Bass, E., and L. Davis. 1988. *The Courage to Heal: A Guide for Women Survivors of Child Sexual Abuse*. New York: Harper and Row.

Courtois, C. 1988. *Healing the Incest Wound: Adult Survivors in Therapy*. New York: W. W. Norton.

Finkelhor, D. 1979. *Sexually Victimized Children*. New York: Free Press.

Herman, J. 1981. *Father-Daughter Incest*. Cambridge, Mass.: Harvard University Press.

Hunter, M. 1990. *Abused Boys: The Neglected Victims of Child Abuse*. New York: Fawcett Columbine.

Maltz, W., and B. Holman. 1990. *Incest and Sexuality: A Guide to Understanding and Healing*. New York: Lexington Books.

Van der Kolk, B. 1986. The psychological consequences of overwhelming life experiences. In *Psychological Trauma*, edited by B. van der Kolk. Washington, D. C.: American Psychiatric Press.

Family Violence and Sexual Assault Bulletin
Family Violence and Sexual Assault Institute
1121 East S.E. Loop, Suite 130
Tyler, TX 75701

Chapter 8

Andrews, G. 1994. *The Treatment of Anxiety Disorders*. London: Cambridge University Press.
This book has an excellent section on social phobias with client manuals and worksheets to help combat such problems.

McKay, M., and M. Davis. 1983. *Messages*. Oakland, Calif.: New Harbinger Publications.
A comprehensive handbook for personal communication.

Zimbardo, P. 1977. *Shyness*. Reading, Mass.: Addison-Wesley.

New Harbinger Publications
Communication Skills Tapes
5674 Shattuck Ave.
Oakland, CA 94609
800-748-6273
New Harbinger cassette titles include: *Making Contact*; *Effective Self-Expression*; *Assertiveness Training*; and *Sexual Communication*. $11.95 each.

Chapter 9

Barbach, L. 1975. *For Yourself: The Fulfillment of Female Sexuality*. New York: Doubleday.

Brooks, G. 1995. *The Centerfold Syndrome: How Men Can Stop Objectifying Women and Achieve True Intimacy*. San Francisco: Jossey-Bass.

Carnes, P. 1992. *Out of the Shadows: Understanding Sexual Addiction*, 2nd ed. Minneapolis: Comp Care.

Carnes, P. 1991. *Don't Call It Love*. New York: Bantam.

Friday, N. 1973. *My Secret Garden: Women's Sexual Fantasies*. New York: Pocket Books.

Hite, S. 1976. *The Hite Report: A Nationwide Study of Female Sexuality*. New York: Dell.

Kitzinger, S. 1986. *Women's Experience of Sex*. New York: Penguin.

Maltz, W., and S. Boss. 1997. *In the Garden of Desire: The Intimate World of Women's Sexual Fantasies — A Journey of Passion, Pleasure, and Self Discovery*. New York: Broadway Books.

McCarthy, B. 1988. *Male Sexual Awareness: Increasing Sexual Satisfaction*. New York: Carroll and Graf.

Steinberg, B., ed. 1992 *The Erotic Impulse*. New York: Putnam.

Zilbergeld, B. 1992. *The New Male Sexuality*. New York: Bantam.

Sex Addicts Anonymous
P. O. Box 3038
Minneapolis, MN 55403
612-871-1520; 612-339-0217

Sex and Love Addicts Anonymous
P. O. Box 119
New Town Branch
Boston, MA 02258
617-332-1845

Chapter 10

Bepko, C. 1997. *The Heart's Progress: A Lesbian Memoir*. New York: Viking.

Brooks, G. 1995. *The Centerfold Syndrome: How Men Can Stop Objectifying Women and Achieve True Intimacy*. San Francisco: Jossey-Bass.

Brooks, G. 1995. Rituals and celebrations in the lives of men. *Newsletter of the Society for the Psychological Study of Men and Masculinity*. (Winter) 1(1):6.

D'Augelli, A., and C. J. Pattterson., eds. 1995. *Lesbian, Gay and Bisexual Identities Over the Lifespan: Psychological Perspectives*. New York: Oxford.

Gagnon, J. H. 1972. The creation of the sexual in early adolescence. In *Twelve to Sixteen: Early Adolescence*, edited by J. Kagan and R. Coles, 231–257. New York: W. W. Norton.

Hunter, M. 1990. *Abused Boys: The Neglected Victims of Child Abuse*. New York: Fawcett Columbine.

Levant, R., with G. Kopecky. 1995. *Masculinity Reconstructed: Changing the Rules of Manhood*. New York: Dutton.

Maltz, W. 1991. *The Sexual Healing Journey*. New York: Harper Collins.

Parrot, A. 1988. *Coping with Date Rape and Aquaintance Rape*. New York: Rosen Publishing.

Resick, P., and M. S. Schnicke. 1992. *Cognitive Processing Therapy for Rape Victims*. Newbury Park, Calif.: Sage.

Steinberg, L., and W. Steinberg. 1995. *Crossing Paths: How Your Child's Adolescence Can Be an Opportunity for Your Own Personal Growth*. New York: Fireside.
This book is a beautifully written discussion of the dynamics between parents and their teenage children.

Westerlund, E. 1992. *Women's Sexuality After Childhood Incest*. New York: Norton.

EMDR Institute
P. O. Box 51010
Pacific Grove, CA 93950-6010
408-372-3900; fax 408-647-9881

Eye Movement Desensitization and Reprocessing (EMDR) is one kind of psychotherapy for dealing specifically with sexual trauma. Contact the above address for referrals to professional therapists trained in EMDR.

National Gay Task Force
1734 14th St. NW
Washington, DC 20009-4309
202-332-6483

Parents and Friends of Lesbians and Gays (PFLAG)
P. O. Box 27605
Washington, DC 20038
203-638-4200

Chapter 11

Jaffe, P., D. Wolfe, and S. Wilson. 1990. *Children of Battered Women*. Newbury Park, Calif.: Sage.

Miller, A. 1983. *For Your Own Good: Hidden Cruelty in Child-rearing and the Roots of Violence*. New York: Farrar, Straus & Giroux.

Pagelow, M. 1984. *Family Violence*. New York: Praeger.

van der Kolk, B. 1986. The psychological consequences of overwhelming life experiences. In *Psychological Trauma*, edited by B. van der Kolk. Washington, D.C.: American Psychiatric Press.

Wolfe, D., L. Zak, S. Wilson, and P. Jaffe. 1986. Child witnesses to violence: Critical issues in behavioral and social adjustment. In *Family Abuse and Its Consequences: New Directions for Research*, edited by G. Hotaling, 228–41. Newbury Park, Calif: Sage.

Family Violence and Sexual Assault Bulletin
Family Violence and Sexual Assault Institute
1121 East S.E. Loop, Suite 130
Tyler, Texas 75701

Additional Resources

For Single Men with Sexual Problems

Barry S. Reynolds, Ph.D.
Human Relations Center
University of Southern California
1002 W. 36th St.
Los Angeles, CA 90089-1591
213-740-6620
Barry Reynolds's tape series, *The Personal Potential Audio Cassette Program for Single Men with Sexual Dysfunction or Relationship Anxiety*, is available for $50.00 plus $7.00 for shipping and handling. I highly recommend it.

For Adult Virgins Who Want to Become Sexual

For Men

Zilbergeld, B. 1992. *The New Male Sexuality*. New York: Bantam.
This book is superb! Along with his coverage of all other aspects of male sexuality, including socialization and self-help for each of the dysfunctions, Zilbergeld writes sensitively and intelligently about male virginity, and provides much information on how to proceed.

Barry S. Reynolds, Ph.D.
Human Relations Center
University of Southern California
1002 W. 36th St.
Los Angeles, CA 90089-1591
213-740-6620

Dr. Barry Reynolds's tape series, *Personal Potential: An Audio Cassette Program for Single Men with Erectile Difficulties, Premature Ejaculation, or Sexual Inexperience and Anxiety* is available for $50.00 plus $7.00 for shipping and handling. This series is an incredible gem, and an unbelievable bargain in my opinion. Reynold uses role playing to tell you what to say and do if your attempts to begin to be sexual are so fraught with anxiety that you cannot perform. In addition the tapes contain men frankly discussing their sexual problems in a group format.

For Women

Heiman, J., and J. Lo Piccolo. 1988. *Becoming Orgasmic: A Sexual and Personal Growth Program for Women*. New York: Fireside.

Kitzinger, S. 1983. *Women's Experience of Sex*. New York: Penguin.

References

Abbey, A., et al. 1996. Alcohol and dating risk factors for sexual assault among college women. *The Psychology of Women Quarterly,* 20(1):147–169.

Ageton, S. 1983. *Sexual Assaults Among Adolescents.* Lexington, Mass.: Heath.

Ainsworth, M. 1982. Attachment: retrospect and prospect. In *The Place of Attachment in Human Behavior,* edited by C. M. Parkes and J. Stevenson-Hinde. 3–30. New York: Basic Books.

Ainsworth, M., M. Blehar, E. Waters, and S. Wall. 1978. *Patterns of Attachment.* Hillsdale, N. J.: Erlbaum.

Alfvin, C. 1995. The Power of Touch. *Women's Day.* May 19, 1995. 92–3.

American Psychiatric Association. 1994. *Diagnostic and Statistical Manual of Mental Disorders,* 4th ed. Washington D. C.: American Psychiatric Association.

Andrews, G., et al. 1994. *The Treatment of Anxiety Disorders.* Cambridge, England: Cambridge University Press.

Barbach, L. 1985. *For Each Other: Sharing Sexual Intimacy.* New York: Anchor.

———. 1975. *For Yourself: The Fulfillment of Female Sexuality.* New York: Signet.

Barlow, D. 1993.*Clinical Handbook of Psychological Disorders.* New York: Guilford.

———. 1988. *Anxiety and Its Disorders: The Nature and Treatment of Anxiety and Panic*. New York: Guilford.

———. 1974. The treatment of sexual deviation: toward a comprehensive behavioral approach. In *Innovative Treatment Methods in Psychopathology*, edited by K. Calhoun, H. Adams, and K. Mitchell. New York: John Wiley and Sons.

Barlow, D., and M. Durand. *Abnormal Psychology*. New York: Brooks/Cole.

Bass, E., and L. Davis. 1988.*The Courage to Heal: A Guide for Women Survivors of Child Sexual Abuse*. New York: Harper and Row.

Beck, A., J. Rush, B. Shaw, and G. Emery. 1979. *Cognitive Therapy of Depression*. New York: Guilford.

Bell, A., and S. Hammersmith. 1978. *Sexual Preference: It's Development in Men and Women*. Bloomington: Indiana University Press.

Bepko, C. 1997. *The Heart's Progress: A Lesbian Memoir*. New York: Viking.

Bolton, F., L. Morris, and A. MacEachron. 1989. *Males at Risk: The Other Side of Child Sexual Abuse*. Newbury Park, Calif.: Sage.

Boston Lesbian Psychologies Collective. 1988. Homophobia: Identifying and treating the oppressor within. *Lesbian Psychologies*. Urbana: University of Illinois Press.

Bowlby, J. 1979. *The Making and Breaking of Affectional Bonds*. London: Tavistock.

———. 1971–79. *Attachment and Loss*, 3 vol. New York: Basic Books.

Branden, N. 1987. *How to Raise Your Self Esteem*. New York: Bantam.

Briere, J. 1996. *Therapy for Adults Molested as Children: Beyond Survival*, 2nd ed. New York: Springer

Brooks, G. 1995. *The Centerfold Syndrome: How Men Can Stop Objectifying Women and Achieve True Intimacy*. San Francisco: Jossey-Bass.

Brown, S. *Treating Adult Children of Alcoholics: A Developmental Perspective*. New York: John Wiley and Sons.

Browne, A. 1993.Violence against women by male partners: prevalence, outcomes, and policy implications. *American Psychologist*. 48(10):1077–87.

———. 1991. The victim's experience: Pathways to disclosure. *Psychotherapy*. (Spring)29(1):1077–87.

Calderone, M. S., and E. Johnson. 1981. *The Family Book About Sexuality.* New York: Harper and Row.

Calderone, M., and J. Ramey. 1982. *Talking with Your Child About Sex.* New York: Random House.

Carnes, P. 1997. *Out of Trauma.* Deerfield Beach, Fla.: Health Communications.

———. 1997. *Sexual Anorexia.* Center City, Minn.: Hazelden Foundation.

———. 1992. *Out of the Shadows: Understanding Sexual Addiction,* 2nd ed. Minneapolis: Comp Care.

———. 1991. *Don't Call It Love.* New York: Bantam.

———. 1990. Sexual addiction. In *The Incest Perpetrator: A Family Member No One Wants to Treat,* edited by A. Horton, B. Johnson, et al. Newbury Park, Calif.: Sage.

———.1988. *Contrary to Love.* Center City, Minn.: Hazelden Foundation.

Cicchetti, D., and V. Carlson, eds. 1989. *Child Maltreatment: Theory and Research on the Causes and Consequences of Child Abuse and Neglect.* New York: Cambridge University Press.

Coopersmith, S. 1967. *The Antecedents of Self-Esteem.* San Francisco: W. H. Freeman and Co.

Courtois, C. 1988. *Healing the Incest Wound: Adult Survivors in Therapy.* New York: W. W. Norton.

Crenshaw, T. J., and J. P. Goldberg. 1996. *Sexual Pharmacology: Drugs that Affect Sexual Function.* New York: Norton.

Crooks, R., and K. Baur. 1993. *Our Sexuality.* Menlo Park, Calif.: Benjamin/Cummings.

Daily, D., ed. 1988. *The Sexually Unusual: A Guide to Helping and Understanding.* New York: Haworth.

D'Augelli, A. R., and C. J. Patterson, eds. 1995. *Lesbian, Gay, and Bisexual Identities Over the Lifespan: Psychological Perspectives.* New York: Oxford University Press.

Davis, M., E. Eshelman, , and M. McKay. 1995.*The Relaxation and Stress Reduction Workbook,* 4th ed. Oakland, Calif.: New Harbinger.

Details. 1993. Generation sex. *Details,* June, 82–99.

DeYoung, M. 1982 *The Sexual Victimization of Children*. Jefferson, N.C.: McFarland.

Donovan, D. M., and D. McIntyre. 1990. *Healing the Hurt Child*. New York: Norton.

Douglas, J., and F. Atwell. 1988. *Love, Intimacy, and Sex*. Thousand Oaks, Calif.: Sage.

Durrell, D. 1989. *Starting Out Right: Essential Parenting Skills for Your Child's First Seven Years*. Oakland, Calif.: New Harbinger.

Ehrenberg, M., and O. Ehrenberg. 1988. *The Intimate Circle: The Sexual Dynamics of Family Life*. New York: Simon and Schuster.

Elium, D., and J. Elium. 1992. *Raising a Son: Parents and the Making of a Healthy Man*. Hillsboro, Ore.: Beyond Words.

Elkind, D. 1981 *The Hurried Child: Growing Up Too Fast Too Soon*. Reading, Mass.: Addison-Wesley.

Erikson, E. 1968. *Identity: Youth and Crisis*. New York: W. W. Norton.

Family Circle. 1994. What stresses you out? *Family Circle*, Feb 1, 8.

Finkelhor, D. 1975. *Sexually Victimized Children*. New York: The Free Press.

Finklehor, D., and L. Baron. 1986. High risk children. In *A Sourcebook on Child Sexual Abuse*, edited by D. Finklehor, 60–88. Beverly Hills, Calif.: Sage.

Finklehor, D., and A. Browne. 1985. The traumatic impact of child sexual abuse: A conceptualization. *American Journal of Orthopsychiatry*. 55: 530–41.

Fisher, H. E. 1993. Love: after all, maybe it's biology. *Psychology Today*. March/April, 40–46, 82.

———. 1992. *Anatomy of Love: The Natural History of Monogamy, Adultery, and Divorce*. New York: W. W. Norton.

Freeman, R. 1988. *BodyLove: Learning to Like Our Looks and Ourselves*. New York: Harper and Row.

Friday, N. 1975. *Forbidden Flowers: More Women's Sexual Fantasies*. New York: Pocket Books.

———. 1973. *My Secret Garden: Women's Sexual Fantasies*. New York: Pocket Books.

Friel, J., and L. Friel. 1988. *Adult Children: The Secrets of Dysfunctional Families*. Deerfield Beach, Fla.: Health Communications.

Gabrino, J., N. Dubrow, K. Kostelny, and C. Pardo. 1992. *Coping with the Consequences of Community Violence*. San Francisco: Jossey-Bass.

Gach, M. 1997. *Acupressure for Lovers: Secrets of Touch for Increasing Intimacy*. New York: Bantam.

Gagnon, J. H. 1972. The creation of the sexual in early adolescence. In *Twelve to sixteen: early adolescence*. edited by J. Kagan, and R. Coles, 231–57. New York: W. W. Norton.

Goldberg, D. 1995. Epidemiology of mental disorders in primary care settings. *Epidemiological Review* 17:182–190.

Golding, J. 1995. Sexual assault history and women's reproductive and sexual health. *Psychology of Women Quarterly* 20(1):101–122.

Goldman, R., and J. Goldman. 1982 *Children's Sexual Thinking*. Boston: Routledge and Kegan Paul.

Goodchilds, J., and G. L. Zellman. 1984. Sexual signaling and sexual aggression in adolescent relationships. In *Pornography and Sexual Aggression*, edited by N. M. Malamuth, and E. Donnerstein, 233–43 Orlando, Fla.: Academic Press.

Gordon, S., and J. Gordon. 1983. *Raising a Child Conservatively in a Sexually Permissive World*. New York: Simon and Schuster.

Green, R. 1974. *Sexual Identity Conflict in Children and Adults*. New York: Basic Books.

Green, R. 1987. *The "Sissy Boy" Syndrome and the Development of Homosexuality*. New Haven, Conn.: Yale University Press.

Greenspan, S. 1985. *First Feelings: Milestones in the Emotional Development of Your Baby and Child from Birth to Four*. New York: Viking.

Harlow, H., and M. Harlow. 1965.The affectional system. In *Advances in the Study of Behavior*, edited by A. M. Schrier, H. F. Harlow, and E. Shore, New York: Academic Press.

———. 1969. Effects of various mother-infant relationships in rhesis mating behavior. In *Determinants of Infant Behavior* IV, edited by B. M. Foss, Amsterdam: Methuen.

Hazan, C., and P. Shaver. 1987. Romantic love conceptualized as an attachment process. *Journal of Personality and Social Psychology*. 52:511–524.

Heiman, J., and J. Lo Piccolo. 1988. *Becoming Orgasmic: A Sexual and Personal Growth Program for Women*. New York: Fireside.

Herman, J. 1992. *Trauma and Recovery*. New York: Basic Books.

———. 1981. *Father-Daughter Incest*. Cambridge: Harvard University Press.

Hite, S. 1976. *The Hite Report: A Nationwwide Study of Feminine Sexuality*. New York: Dell.

Horton, A., et al. 1990. *The Incest Perpetrator: A Family Member No One Wants to Treat*. Newbury Park, Calif.: Sage.

Horton, P., H. Gerwitz, and K. Kreutter. 1988. *The Solace Paradigm*. Madison, Conn.: International Universities Press.

Hunt, M. 1974. *Sexual Behavior in the 1970's*. Chicago: Playboy Press.

Hunter, M. 1990. *Abused Boys: The Neglected Victims of Child Abuse*. New York: Fawcett Columbine.

Hutchinson, M. 1985. *Transforming Body Image: Learning to Love the Body You Have*. Freedom, Calif.: The Crossing Press.

Intons-Peterson, M. J. 1988. *Children's Concept of Gender*. Norwood, N. J.: Ablex Publishing.

Jaffe, P., D. Wolfe, and S. Wilson. 1990. *Children of Battered Women: Issues in Child Development and Intervention Planning*. Newbury Park, Calif.: Sage.

Kinsey, A., W. Pomeroy, and C. Martin. 1948. *Sexual Behavior in the Human Male*. Philadelphia: Saunders.

Kinsey, A., W. Pomeroy, C. Martin, and P. Gebhard. 1953. *Sexual Behavior in the Human Female*. Philadelphia: Saunders.

Kirk, C. 1993. *Leaving Abusive Partners*. Newbury Park, Calif.: Sage.

Kitzinger, S. 1983. *Woman's Experience of Sex*. New York: Penguin.

Korn, D. L. 1997. Clinical applications of EMDR in treating survivors of sexual abuse. Paper presented to the 1997 EMDR International Association Conference, San Francisco.

Koss, M., C. Gidycz, and N. Wisniewski. 1987. The scope of rape: incidence and prevalence of sexual aggression and victimization in a national sample of higher education students. *Journal of Consulting and Clinical Psychology* 55:162–70.

Koss, M. P. 1988. Hidden rape: sexual aggression and victimization in a national sample in higher education. In *Rape and Sexual Assault,* edited by A. Burgess, 11:3–25. New York: Garland Press.

Koss, M., and M. Harvey. 1991. *The Rape Victim: Clinical and Community Interventions.* 2nd ed. Newbury Park, Calif.: Sage.

Lazarus, A. 1988. A multimodal perspective on problems of sexual desire. In *Sexual Desire Disorders,* edited by S. Lieblum and R. Rosen, 145–67. New York: Guilford.

———. 1978. Overcoming sexual inadequacy. In *The Handbook of Sex Therapy,* edited by J. LoPiccolo and L. LoPiccolo, 19–34. New York: Plenum.

———. 1971. *Behavior Therapy and Beyond.* New York: McGraw-Hill.

Laufer, M. 1976. The central masturbation fantasy: the final sexual organization, and adolescence. *The Psychoanalytic Study of the Child* 31: 297–316.

Leight, L. 1988. *Raising Sexually Healthy Children.* New York: Rawson Associates.

Levant, R., with G. Kopecky. 1995. *Masculinity Reconstructed: Changing the Rules of Manhood.* New York: Dutton.

Levant, R., and W. Pollack. 1996. *A New Psychology of Men.* New York: Basic Books.

Levine, S. B. 1988. Intrapsychic and individual aspects of sexual desire. In *Sexual Desire Disorders,* edited by S. Lieblum, and R. Rosen, New York: Guilford.

Levy, B. 1991. *Dating Violence: Young Women in Danger.* Seattle, Wash.: Seal Press.

Lewis, H., and M. Lewis. 1983. *Sex Education Begins at Home: How to Raise Sexually Healthy Children.* Norwalk, Conn.: Appleton-Century-Crofts.

Lieblum, S., and R. Rosen, eds. 1989. *Principles and Practice of Sex Therapy,* 2nd ed. New York: Guilford.

Lobel, K,. ed. 1986. *Naming the Silence: Speaking Out About Lesbian Battering.* Seattle Wash.: Seal Press.

McCarthy, B. 1988. *Male Sexual Awareness: Increasing Sexual Satisfaction.* New York: Carroll and Graf.

McCarthy, B., and E. McCarthy. 1989. *Female Sexual Awareness: Achieving Sexual Fulfillment*. New York: Carroll and Graf.

McKay, M., and P. Fanning. 1992. *Self-Esteem*. Oakland, Calif.: New Harbinger.

McKay, M., P. Rogers, and J. McKay. 1989. *When Anger Hurts: Quieting the Storm Within*. Oakland, Calif.: New Harbinger.

McGoldrick, M. 1982. Irish Families. In *Ethnicity and Family Therapy*, edited by McGoldrick, et al., 310–39. New York: Guilford.

Madaras, L. 1988. *The What's Happening to My Body Book for Boys*. New York: New Market Press.

Maltz, W. 1991. *The Sexual Healing Journey: A Guide for Survivors of Sexual Abuse*. New York: Harper Collins.

Maltz, W., and S. Boss. 1997. *In the Garden of Desire: The Intimate World of Women's Sexual Fantasies—A Journey of Passion, Pleasure, and Self Discovery*. New York: Broadway Books.

Maltz, W., and B. Holman. 1987. *Incest and Sexuality: A Guide to Understanding and Healing*. New York: Lexington Books.

Markway, B., C. Carmin, A. Pollard, T. Flynn. 1992. *Dying of Embarrassment: Help for Social Anxiety and Phobia*. Oakland, Calif.: New Harbinger.

Masters, W., V. Johnson, and R. Kolodny. 1975. *Human Sexuality*. Boston: Little Brown.

Miller, A. 1983. *For Your Own Good: Hidden Cruelty in Child-Rearing and the Roots of Violence*. New York: Farrar, Strauss & Giroux.

Moitoza, E. 1982. Portugese families. In *Ethnicity and Family Therapy*, edited by McGoldrick, et al., 412–37. New York: Guilford.

Money, J. 1980. *Love and Love Sickness: The Science of Sex, Gender Difference, and Pair Bonding*. Baltimore: Johns Hopkins Press.

Money, J., and A. Ehrhardt. 1972. *Man and Woman: Boy and Girl*. Baltimore: Johns Hopkins Press.

Montagu, A. 1971. *Touching: The Human Significance of the Skin*. New York: Columbia University Press.

Muehlenhard, C. 1989. Young men pressured into having sex with women. *Medical Aspects of Human Sexuality*. (April):50–62.

———. 1988. Misinterpreting dating behavior and the risk of date rape. *Journal of Social and Clinical Psychology*. 6:20–37.

Muehlenhard, C., and M. Linton. 1987. Date rape and sexual aggression in dating situations: incidence and risk factors. *Journal of Consulting Psychology* 54:872–879.

Muehlenhard, C., and J. Schrag. 1991. Nonviolent sexual coercion. *Acquaintance Rape: The Hidden Crime*. New York: Wiley.

Nelson, J. B. 1983. *Between Two Gardens: Reflections on Sexuality and Religious Experience*. New York: Pilgrim..

Olweus, D. 1993. *Bullying at School: What We Know and What We Can Do*. Cambridge, Mass.: Blackwell Publishers.

Pagelow, M. 1984. *Family Violence*. New York: Praeger.

Parrot, A. 1988. *Coping with Date Rape and Acquaintance Rape*. New York: Rosen Publishing.

Pierce, L., and R. Pierce. 1990. Adolescent / sibling incest perpetrators, In *The Incest Perpetrator: A Family Member No One Wants to Treat*, edited by A. Horton, et al., 99–107. Newbury Park, Calif.: Sage.

Pleck, J., and J. Sawyer, eds. 1974. *Men and Masculinity*. New Jersey: Prentice-Hall.

Polonsky, D. 1995. *Talking About Sex*. Washington D. C.: American Psychiatric Press.

Potter-Efron, R. 1994. *Angry All the Time: An Emergency Guide to Anger Control*. Oakland, Calif.: New Harbinger.

Ratner, E. 1990. *The Other Side of the Family*. Deerfield Beach, Fla.: Health Communications.

Reinisch, J., L. Rosenblum, S. Sanders, eds. 1987. *Masculinity/Femininity: Basic Perspectives*. New York: Oxford University Press.

Reinisch, J. 1990. *The Kinsey Institute New Report on Sex*. New York: St. Martin's Press.

Resick, P., and M. Schnicke. 1993. *Cognitive Processing for Rape Victims*. Newbury Park, Calif.: Sage.

Richards, L., B. Rollerson, and J. Phillips. 1991. Perceptions of submissiveness: implications for victimization. *The Journal of Psychology* 125: 407–411.

Rosen, R., and S. Lieblum. 1992. *Erectile Disorders: Assessment and Treatment*. New York: Guilford.

———. 1987. Current approaches to the evaluation of sexual desire disorders. *Journal of Sex Research* 23(2):141–62.

Ross, M., and W. Arrindell. 1988. Perceived parental rearing patterns of homosexual and heterosexual men. *Journal of Sex Research* 24:275–81.

Scharff, D. 1982. *The Sexual Relationship: An Object Relations View of the Family*. Boston: Routledge and Kegan Paul.

Shapiro, F. 1995. *Eye Movement Desensitization and Reprocessing: Basic Principles, Protocols, and Procedures*. New York: Guilford.

———. 1989. Efficacy of the eye movement desensitization method in the treatment of traumatic memories. *Journal of Traumatic Stress* 2:199–223.

Shaver, P., and C. Hazan. 1993. Adult romantic attachment: theory and empirical evidence. In *Advances in Personal Relationships*, edited by D. Perlman and W. Jones, 4:29–70. Greenwich, Conn.: JAI Press.

Shaver, P., C. Hazan, and D. Bradshaw. 1988. Love as attachment: The integration of three behavioral systems. In *The Psychology of Love*, edited by R. Sternberg, and M. Barnes, 68–99. New Haven, Conn.: Yale University Press.

———. 1984. Infant-caretaker attachment and adult romantic love: similarities and differences, continuities and discontinuities. Paper presented at 2nd International Conference on Personal Relationships, Madison,Wisc.

Smyth, L. 1995. *A Clinician's Manual for the Cognitive-Behavioral Treatment of Posttraumatic Stress Disorder*. Harve de Grace, Md.: RTR Publishing.

Starr, R., and D. Wolfe, eds. 1991. *The Effects of Child Abuse and Neglect*. New York: Guilford.

Steinbaum, E. 1994. Image problem: Why our children think their bodies will never measure up. *The Boston Globe Magazine*, October 16, 18–24.

Steinberg, B., ed. 1992. *The Erotic Impulse*. New York: Putnam.

Steinberg, L., and A. Levine. 1990. *You and Your Adolescent*. New York: Harper Perennial.

Steinberg, L., and W. Steinberg. 1995. *Crossing Paths: How Your Child's Adolescence Can Be an Opportunity for Your Own Personal Growth*. New York: Fireside.

Storms, M. 1980. Theories of sexual orientation. *Journal of Personality and Social Psychology* 38:783–92.

Strauss, M., R. Gelles, and S. Steinmetz. 1980. *Behind Closed Doors: Violence in the American Family.* Garden City, N. Y.: Anchor Press, Doubleday.

Tiefer, L. 1995. *Sex Is Not a Natural Function.* New York: Westview Press.

———. 1979. *Human Sexuality: Feelings and Functions.* New York: Harper and Row.

Treadway, D. 1989. *Before It's Too Late: Working with Substance Abuse in the Family.* New York: Norton.

van der Kolk, B. 1987. *Psychological Trauma.* Washington, D. C.: American Psychiatric Press.

van der Kolk, B., A. McFarlane, and L. Weisaeth. 1996. *Traumatic Stress: The Effects of Overwhelming Experience on Mind, Body and Society.* New York: Guilford.

Vaughan, K., M. Armstrong, R. Gold, N. O'Connor, et al. 1994 . A trial of eye movement desensitization compared to image habituation training and applied muscle relaxation in post traumatic stress disorder. *Journal of Behavior Therapy and Experimental Psychiatry* 25:283–91.

Von Korff, M., S. Shapiro, J. D. Burke, et al. 1987. Anxiety and depression in primary care clinics: comparison of diagnostic interview schedule, general health questionnarie, and practitioner assessment. *Archives of General Psychiatry* 44:152–156.

Walker, L. 1991. Post-traumatic stress disorder in women: diagnosis and treatment of battered women syndrome. *Psychotherapy* 28(1):21–29.

———. 1984. *The Battered Woman Syndrome.* New York: Springer.

Wallach, L. B. 1993. Helping children cope with violence. *Young Children,* 48(4):4–ll.

Welts, E. 1982. Greek families. In *Ethnicity and Family Therapy,* edited by McGoldrick, et al., 269–88. New York: Guilford.

Westerlund, E. 1992. *Women's Sexuality After Childhood Incest.* New York: Norton.

Westra, B., and H. Martin. 1981. Children of battered women. *Maternal-Child Nursing Journal* 10:41–54.

Whitfield, C. L. 1987. *Healing the Child Within*. Deerfield Beach, Fla.: Health Communications.

Whitam, F. 1980. The prehomosexual male child in three societies: The United States, Guatamala, Brazil. *Archives of Sexual Behavior* 9:89–99.

Williams, L. M., and D. Finklehor. 1988. The characteristics of incestuous fathers: a review of recent studies. In *The Handbook of Sexual Assault: Issues, Theories, and Treatment of the Offender*, edited by W. L. Marshall, D. R. Laws, and H. E. Barbaree, New York: Plenum.

Wolf, N. 1991. *The Beauty Myth*. New York: William Morrow.

Wolf, S. 1993. *Guerilla Dating Tactics*. New York: Dutton.

Wolf, S. 1988. A model of sexual aggression/addiction. In *The Sexually Unusual: A Guide to Understanding and Helping*, edited by D. Daily, 131–37. New York: Haworth.

Wolfe, D. A., P. Jaffe, S. Wilson, and L. Zak. 1988. A multivariate investigaation of children's adjustment to family violence. In *Family Abuse and Its Consequences: New Directions for Research*, edited by G. Hotaling, 228–41. Newbury Park, Calif.: Sage.

Wolfe, D. A., L. Zak, S. Wilson, and P. Jaffe. 1986. Child witnesses to violence: critical issues in behavioral and social adjustment. *Journal of Abnormal Child Psychology*: 14:95–104.

Young, J. 1994. *Cognitive Therapy for Personality Disorders: A Schema-Focused Approach*. Sarasota, Fla.: Professional Resource.

Zilbergeld, B. 1992. *The New Male Sexuality*. New York: Bantam.

Zimbardo, P. 1977. *Shyness*. Reading, Mass.: Addison Wesley.